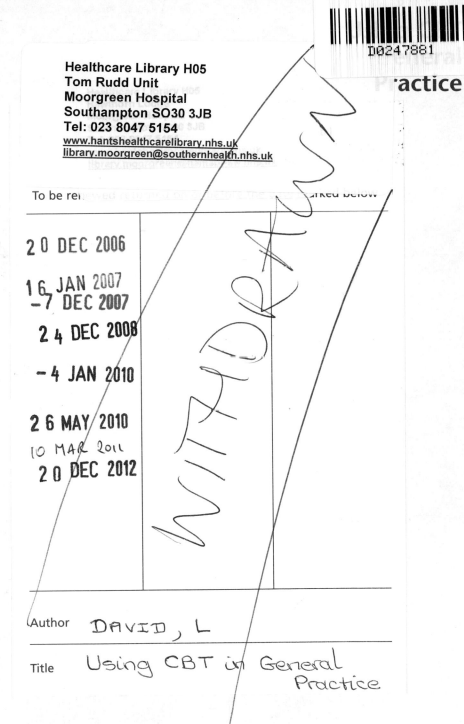

Author DAVID, L

Title Using CBT in General Practice

Using CBT in General Practice

The 10 Minute Consultation

Lee David

MB BS, BSc, MRCGP, MA in cognitive behavioural therapy
GP and Cognitive Behavioural Therapist, Hertfordshire

Scion

© Scion Publishing Ltd, 2006
First published 2006

A CIP catalogue record for this book is available from the British Library.

ISBN 1 904842 33 X

Scion Publishing Limited
Bloxham Mill, Barford Road, Bloxham, Oxfordshire OX15 4FF
www.scionpublishing.com

Important Note from the Publisher

The information contained within this book was obtained by Scion Publishing Limited from sources believed by us to be reliable. However, while every effort has been made to ensure its accuracy, no responsibility for loss or injury whatsoever occasioned to any person acting or refraining from action as a result of information contained herein can be accepted by the author or publishers.

The reader should remember that medicine is a constantly evolving science and while the authors and publishers have ensured that all dosages, applications and practices are based on current indications, there may be specific practices which differ between communities. You should always follow the guidelines laid down by the manufacturers of specific products and the relevant authorities in the country in which you are practising.

Typeset by Phoenix Photosetting, Chatham, Kent, UK
Printed by Biddles Ltd, King's Lynn, UK, www.biddles.co.uk

Contents

Foreword: A GP's wish list

I wish there were 48 hours in the day, and that I needed no sleep, or holidays, or family time; because then I could spend as much time with every patient as they needed.

I wish I only needed to be told something once, and that I remembered everything I *was* told, and that – amongst everything I was told – I could always tell what is important from what is not; because then I could incorporate all the important things into my everyday practice.

I wish I could endlessly acquire new skills, and be ever eager for new responsibilities, and have access to unlimited resources; because then I wouldn't feel threatened by a rising tide of expectation.

I wish it were better understood that there's more to general practice than following every protocol, and obeying every guideline, and ticking every box; because then I should feel more comfortable with tailoring what I offer to the personal circumstances of individual patients.

I wish it were easier to accept that patients are allowed to present with unhappiness and worries, or with bad habits and irrational behaviour, or to be irritating and frustrating; because then I could learn how to help them effectively without feeling too many twinges of resentment.

I wish more GPs could share the fulfilment that some of their colleagues derive from undertaking Balint work, or counselling, or family therapy; because then they'd more often have the satisfaction of knowing they personally can make a lasting difference in a patient's life.

I wish more GPs appreciated that CBT is a fast, effective and easy to learn way of making this sort of difference in patients' lives; because then they'd want to try it for themselves.

I wish everybody knew that you don't necessarily have to be a specialist in CBT in order to practise it effectively; because then more GPs would want to add it to their repertoire and use it in their routine consultations.

I wish Lee David's book had been around 20 years ago; because then I could have helped a lot more people and had a lot more fun.

I wish every GP would read it; because then *they'd* be able to help a lot more people and have a lot more fun.

Roger Neighbour MA DSc FRCP PRCGP
Bedmond, Herts
July 2006

Preface

Using CBT in General Practice is a practical introduction to cognitive-behavioural approaches to consulting in primary care. It provides an overview of the basic principles of cognitive-behavioural therapy (CBT) and outlines a simple method of using these principles in 10-minute consultations. It shows how CBT can be used to improve the management of many common primary care problems, including emotional disorders and psychological difficulties associated with chronic physical disease.

This book is aimed at general practitioners (GPs), but is also highly relevant to a wide range of other health professionals who have a role in promoting the emotional well-being of patients in primary care, including practice nurses, health visitors, counsellors, community psychiatric nurses and occupational therapists. For the sake of simplicity, I have used the term 'GP' throughout the book.

CBT is one of the most effective psychological treatments for many common mental health problems. Such difficulties make up a significant portion of the primary care workload, but most regions have little or no access to CBT services for the vast majority of patients.

As a GP myself, I fully appreciate the enormous challenges and pressures of working in primary care. When I undertook post-graduate training in CBT, I was struck by how valuable the training was to my practice as a GP. I also discovered that, as a GP, I *already* possessed many of the skills required for effective CBT.

As a consequence, I developed an innovative approach to teaching CBT to other primary care health professionals, which was specifically designed to be used within 'real-life' setting of primary care (David and Freeman, 2006). The feedback from these courses has shown that simple perspectives and concepts from CBT *can* be effective and useful within routine GP appointments.

I also discovered that, as well as helping patients, CBT offers a practical and useful method for GPs to:

- Cope better with 'heartsink' experiences
- Reduce stress and burnout
- Use as a tool to reflect upon difficult consultations
- Use for teaching, training and mentoring

This book offers a practical and realistic method of using CBT principles within routine, time-limited primary care appointments. It was specifically written with the needs of busy GPs in mind.

Lee David
May 2006

Acknowledgements

I would like to thank a number of people for their support in writing this book.

My thanks go to Professor George Freeman for his invaluable ongoing support in the dvelopment of the 'CBM' approach. I would also like to thank all GP participants at '10-minute CBT' training events, whose participation, feedback and enthusiasm have contributed to the development of this book. I am also greatly indebted to a number of colleagues who kindly read and commented on the manuscript of this book. In particular, thanks go to Ruth Danson, Clare Etherington and Arti Maini.

I am very grateful to Scion Publishing, and in particular, my editor Jonathan Ray, for their support during the writing of this book.

I must also thank all the patients that I have worked with using CBT. The success of CBT techniques depends upon individual patients' own commitment and work, often during very challenging circumstances. I feel privileged to have been able to share the CBT approach and to have been part of each person's individual life journey.

Finally, my greatest thanks must go to my family, especially my parents, Cat and George, whose support, love and belief in me has been central to the writing of this book, as with all my achievements in life.

Introduction

How to Use this Book

Using CBT in General Practice is divided into three sections:

- Section A is an introduction to the theory and application of cognitive-behavioural approaches in the primary care setting.
- Section B introduces some more advanced techniques and theory of CBT, including an overview of problem-solving therapy.
- Section C is a clinical reference section. Each chapter provides an overview of a common psychological disorder and describes a cognitive-behavioural approach to helping patients with the problem.

It is particularly important for readers to learn and develop their skills and understanding of CBT, not simply by reading this book, but through *practice*. To facilitate this 'hands-on' learning, a variety of practical exercises have been included in most chapters. This will help readers to incorporate CBT theory into their own practice.

It is not necessary to work through all the chapters in order. As you progress through Section A, for example, you may develop questions about particular patients or clinical disorders. In this case, it can be helpful to flip to Section C, to understand the specific approach to a particular condition.

Overview of Chapters

Section A: Introduction to CBT

Chapter 1 sets the scene for the book, by looking at what CBT has to offer general practice. This chapter also explores the relationship between CBT, patient-centred consulting and narrative-based care.

Chapter 2 explores how cognitive-behavioural approaches can be adapted for use in GP consultations and introduces the reader to the 'cognitive-behavioural model' (CBM).

Chapter 3 introduces some basic principles and theory of CBT. It uses practical examples to illustrate relationships between thoughts, emotions, physical feelings, behaviour and environmental factors.

Chapter 4 is a practical guide to using a cognitive-behavioural approach within primary care appointments. It covers what to ask and how to elicit relevant information from patients.

Chapter 5 is a key chapter which gives an overview of the consultation and communication skills that are essential to effectively use CBT in practice.

Section B: Further principles of CBT

Chapter 6 introduces a way of understanding GPs' own difficulties in coping with difficult consultations or 'heartsink' patients.

Chapter 7 outlines some approaches in helping patients to cope with negative thoughts. This includes ways to challenge and 'reframe' unhelpful thoughts and beliefs.

Chapter 8 looks at how to promote changes in unhelpful behaviour – a key factor in the 'vicious cycles' that often maintain or worsen problems.

Chapter 9 gives an overview of how to solve any practical life problems that may be contributing to emotional distress.

Chapter 10 looks at some of the deeper thought processes which may underlie problems: 'core beliefs' and 'rules for living'. These are illustrated using difficulties that GPs may experience when consulting.

Section C: Clinical applications of CBT

This section contains clinical reference chapters which provide an overview of a range of common clinical conditions and problems:

Chapter 11: Anxiety and panic disorder

Chapter 12: Depression

Chapter 13: Low self-esteem

Chapter 14: Health anxiety and hypochondriasis

Chapter 15: Psychological aspects of chronic disease

Chapter 16: Additional reading and website resources, including useful 'self-help' information for patients and suggestions for further CBT training. *References* are grouped into sections, to help the reader identify further information/reading on specific topics. Each section is listed alphabetically. This includes all references quoted within the text, as well as a range of other books and journal articles used in writing this book.

About the Author

After training as a GP on the Oxford vocational training scheme, I undertook a two-year, part-time course at the University of Wales, which led to a Masters in Cognitive-Behavioural Counselling in December 2004.

Since then, I have split my week between working as a part-time GP and as a 'standard' cognitive-behavioural therapist.

I also have a particular interest in teaching and have developed an innovative method of teaching GPs and other primary care practitioners how to improve their consultations using basic principles of CBT. I run workshops for a wide variety of primary care educational groups throughout the UK.

Chapter 1

Setting the scene: understanding what CBT can offer

- CBT approaches offer a useful and effective addition to GPs' existing 'toolkit' of skills

- Simple CBT approaches can be used within a 10-minute consultation

- GPs *already* possess many of the skills required to learn and use CBT in their consultations

- The cognitive-behavioural model (CBM) offers a useful self-reflective tool for GPs

Background

Psychological symptoms and distress are widespread and prevalent in primary care. Worry, tiredness and sleepless nights affect more than half of adults at some time, and as many as 15% of the UK population experience some form of diagnosable neurotic disorder (Craig & Boardman, 1997). Anxiety and depression, often occurring together, are the most commonly seen emotional disorders in general practice.

Overall, about one-quarter of GP consultations are for patients with mental disorders, who consult about twice as often as other patients (Craig & Boardman, 1997). However, time constraints and competing priorities frequently limit a GP's ability to help these patients.

Why learn about CBT?

CBT strategies offer an effective approach to the management of a wide variety of psychological and emotional disorders, including depression, generalized anxiety disorder, panic attacks, social phobia, obsessive–compulsive disorder, and health anxiety. It is also useful for many physical disorders including diabetes, epilepsy, chronic pain, irritable bowel syndrome and insomnia (Enright, 1997; DOH, 2001).

The important role of CBT in the management of depression and anxiety has been highlighted by guidelines issued by the National Institute of Clinical Excellence (NICE, 2004a). This may be particularly important for patients with mild to moderate symptoms, where there is far less evidence of the benefit of medication such as antidepressants.

CBT techniques are also likely to prove popular with patients, who often prefer psychological approaches to their problems. Many patients are sceptical of the benefits of drug treatment, preferring approaches such as counselling or complementary therapies (Kadam *et al.*, 2001).

However, whilst there is a clear need for CBT services, *access* to CBT remains limited or even non-existent for many primary care patients. GPs cannot be expected to fill this gap, but specific skills and techniques from CBT *can* offer a way of improving GPs' management of many common general practice problems.

Such training fits within the spectrum of CBT-based interventions, including 'standard' CBT, computerized CBT and self-help literature based on CBT principles ('bibliotherapy').

Reminders: Why learn about CBT?

- Emotional disorders are widespread and common in primary care
- CBT is an evidence-based treatment for many psychological disorders including depression and anxiety
- Psychological approaches are popular with patients
- There is limited access to CBT services in many parts of the UK

Using CBT in primary care consultations

Although CBT traditionally involves 6–20 one-hour sessions with patients, some basic principles and techniques of CBT can also be applied effectively within the context of 10-minute primary care consultations.

This book presents a specifically designed approach to applying CBT within routine, time-limited GP consultations. This involves using a 'cognitive-behavioural model' (CBM) to understand and overcome patients' psychological and emotional difficulties (see *Box 1.1*).

Box 1.1:
Features of the
CBM approach

- Primary aim is to *enhance understanding* of problems from a cognitive-behavioural viewpoint
- Flexible, generic model, useful within a variety of practice settings and for many common primary care problems
- Enhances effective use of limited consultation time
- Simple model – avoids excessive theory or jargon
- Useful for psychological aspects of physical disorders as well as mental health problems
- Encourages patients to take responsibility for problems
- Useful for reflection and stress management of GPs

A new consultation model for general practice

Communication has been increasingly acknowledged as the cornerstone of effective consulting in primary care. Consequently, a diverse range of consultation models for general practice has developed, arising from a variety of backgrounds. GP consultations have been evaluated from perspectives as diverse as psychotherapy (Balint, 1964), transactional analysis (Berne, 1964) and medical anthropology (Helman, 1990).

The CBM also contributes to improving effective communication and consulting within primary care. It provides a new theoretical framework for making sense of problems, based on CBT theory. This new way to 'conceptualize' difficulties can make them easier to understand and can help to identify new coping strategies or solutions for problems.

Enhancing patient-centred consulting

In recent years, particular attention has been given to the concept of patient-centred consulting, although as yet there is no consensus on a definition for this process. However, there is a considerable body of literature emphasizing the need to understand patients' experiences of primary care consultations and of their illness/problems, as well as exploring ways to achieve this. For example, Becker and Maiman's (1975) 'health belief model' defined the need to take into account patients' 'ideas, concerns and expectations' about their illness. Pendleton *et al.* (1984) defined seven tasks to be tackled in a consultation, which include defining the patient's reason(s) for attendance, achieving a shared understanding of the problem(s) and sharing decision-making by GP and patient about management options.

The CBM provides a unique method of conceptualizing any problem, emotional reaction or situation from *the perspective of the individual patient*. For example, two patients with very similar symptoms may have entirely different underlying thoughts and fears. One person with panic attacks might dread a medical catastrophe ("I might have a heart attack and die"), whereas another fears looking foolish in public ("I will look like a fool and lose the respect of my colleagues").

Achieving a shared understanding of a problem(s) using the CBM involves both GP and patient developing insight into issues from a cognitive-behavioural perspective. Patient-centredness in this context involves seeking to understand the specific and unique thoughts, feelings and behaviours that comprise any individual patient's reaction to events. Identifying these can help the patient to make sense of problems, and promotes an increased sense of control over difficulties in addition to helping identify useful, new coping strategies and solutions.

Focusing on consultation skills

Learning and practicing core consultation skills for the CBM is an important way for GPs to learn how to effectively implement cognitive-behavioural skills in routine practice. These skills are outlined in *Box 1.2*.

Box 1.2: Core consultation skills for the CBM (see also Chapter 5)

- Agenda setting
- Focused approach: stay specific and concrete
- Cognitive empathy
- Collaboration and guided discovery
- Obtaining feedback from patients
- Link-making
- Setting and reviewing homework

These consultation skills are derived from core communication skills used when training cognitive-behavioural therapists. It is also important to note that many GPs *already* possess many of these skills. For example, listening empathically, summarizing and obtaining feedback from patients by checking their understanding of the consultation may be commonplace in many primary care consultations. Other skills, such as 'focusing on the concrete' and 'guided discovery', may be less familiar to many GPs.

There is some crossover between the skills identified by the CBM and those of existing GP consultation models. For example, 'summarization' is a key concept defined by Neighbour (1987; see *Box 1.3*) and is also central to the CBM. Similarly, his concept of 'hand-over' reflects the skill of collaboration. Neighbour (1992) also described a process of 'Socratic questioning' for facilitating learning in trainee GPs, which is closely related to the 'guided discovery' of the CBM.

Box 1.3: Five process for effective consulting (Neighbour, 1987)

- **Connecting:** skills in building rapport
- **Summarizing:** listening and eliciting skills to facilitate effective assessment
- **Hand-over:** communicating skills to hand-over responsibility for management
- **Safety-netting:** predicting skills to suggest contingency plan for worst scenario
- **Housekeeping:** self-awareness to clear mind of psychological remains of one consultation so it has no detrimental effect on the next

Learning to develop highly collaborative relationships with patients is a key skill needed to implement cognitive behavioural approaches effectively in practice. The concept of collaboration parallels those of shared decision-making and doctor–patient partnership, and is likely to promote patient-centred consultations.

The CBM defines several methods of developing collaboration, including: by negotiating an agenda at the beginning of consultations, by actively obtaining patient feedback, by giving copies of written records of consultations to patients, and through the use of 'guided discovery'. Here, clinicians use specific questions and reflective statements to help patients identify and make links between psychological, physical and environmental factors *for themselves*.

Reminders: The CBM – a new consultation model for general practice

- The CBM is a method of using CBT theory to improve GP consultations
- The model provides a framework for understanding problems in terms of the unique thoughts, feelings and behaviours in any individual reaction to events
- Using the CBM promotes a patient-centred approach, through consultation skills such as agenda-setting, collaboration and obtaining feedback
- GPs *already* possess many of the key skills needed to incorporate CBT-based approaches into consultations

Enhancing a narrative-based approach to consultations

Mental health care in general practice includes a varied spectrum of patients. The majority of these patients experience mild to moderate symptoms and distress and are managed solely within the primary care setting. Such patients may be difficult to define according to diagnostic labels such as those described by DSM-IV (APA, 1994) but are still in need of effective help and support with their difficulties.

This difficulty is highlighted by supporters of a narrative-based approach to primary care (Bracken & Thomas, 2001; Launer, 2002), who suggest that diagnostic labels, such as 'depression' or 'post-traumatic stress disorder', may 'pathologize' many people who are simply struggling with adverse life experiences (Heath, 1999; Middleton & Shaw, 2000). These labels may not fit the complex nature of many people's problems and the varied ways in which they may present to primary care (Armstrong, 1996).

A narrative approach listens to the 'story' of each patient's unique experience, whilst leaving open the possibility that conventional diagnostic labels such as 'depression' may or may not be useful in various circumstances. This can help patients to make sense of their experiences and explore their *own* preferred options for change.

The central concept of the CBM is to discover the detailed and in-depth *narratives* of patients' unique experiences. The CBM can be a very powerful way of telling the 'story' of patients' problems, often with more detail and in greater depth than patients may spontaneously offer. Effective use of the model effectively does not rely on the presence of diagnostic labels, although using it to explore difficulties may also improve diagnosis of 'hidden' psychological problems such as depression.

The CBM provides a structure for making sense of problems from a new perspective and promotes an increased sense of control over difficulties. This enables patients to disentangle themselves from their 'stories' and may identify ways to 'rewrite' future narratives by finding appropriate, new coping strategies and solutions for problems.

Reminders: CBT and narrative approaches

- Diagnostic labels do not always fit patients' complex problems and experiences
- CBT does not rely on diagnostic labels for effectiveness
- A narrative approach attempts to discover the 'story' of each patient's unique experience
- The CBM helps patients express a detailed narrative of their experiences from a cognitive-behavioural perspective
- The CBM can help patients to 'rewrite' future narratives

Benefits from learning cognitive-behavioural approaches

Even within 10-minute consultations, cognitive-behavioural approaches can be very useful for both health professionals and patients. Learning to use the CBM can increase a clinician's confidence and skills in discussing psychological issues, making consultations more interesting and enjoyable. This enhances personal and job satisfaction, and can also improve both recognition and management of disorders such as anxiety and depression.

The CBM provides a structured approach that helps to make sense of complex information about psychological and physical problems. This can improve the management of these problems and may make such consultations feel less overwhelming or stressful for GPs.

The CBM approach encourages patients to take responsibility for understanding and managing their own problems (patient empowerment). Using CBT-based approaches may also markedly improve some patients' symptoms. This may arise through patients' improved understanding of the nature of their problems as well as from the use of simple cognitive or behavioural treatment strategies.

Using the CBM can improve the relationship between GP and patient. The deeper understanding of the patient gained by using the CBM to explore problems can increase a clinician's empathy for patients. This itself may encourage more positive attitudes and improve difficult relationships with certain patients. The CBM also offers useful strategies to improve the management of 'heartsink' patients. This includes using the model to reflect on a GP's *own* negative and unhelpful reactions to such patients.

Finally, the CBM is a particularly useful technique to help GPs improve personal difficulties such as stress, anxiety, low mood and irritability. It can also be an extremely helpful approach to clinical supervision, mentoring or teaching and training. Self-reflection using CBM approaches can be an extremely powerful and useful tool for both experienced and new GPs alike.

Box 1.4:
Summary of benefits from use of cognitive-behavioural approaches

Benefits for GPs
- Increases confidence and ability to diagnose and manage psychological disorders
- Provides a structure to manage complex information in consultations
- Enhances job satisfaction – consultations more interesting and enjoyable
- Improves time management – make more effective use of time
- New skills for approaching problems, including simple cognitive and behavioural strategies
- Helps understand and improve relationships with patients, including 'heartsink' patients

continued

Box 1.4:
continued

- Useful for coping with a GP's own difficulties and problems
- Also useful for teaching, mentoring, clinical supervision and self-reflection

Benefits for patients
- Helps patients to understand and make sense of their problems
- Improves relationships with health professionals – patients may feel better understood and listened to
- Aids discovery of new coping strategies or solutions to problems
- Reduces some distressing emotions and symptoms
- Empowers patients to cope with problems themselves

Can CBT *really* be used in 10 minute GP consultations?

I believe that the answer to this question is '**Yes**'! The CBM approach *can* and *is* being used effectively by many GPs and other health professionals in primary care. These skills can be acquired from brief workshops and through reading and practising self-reflective learning.

I will leave the last words to some of the GP participants from our CBM workshops, who describe how they used the CBM approach in a variety of 'real-life' consultations:

Female GP, London

"*A patient experienced… panic attacks over a few years… basically we tried to explore… how he was responding to a panic attack, what was his reaction to it and whether there was any trigger that he was unaware of… We managed to find out that there was a relationship between things happening at work and the panic attacks and also the way he actually was dealing with [them] was probably causing [more] anxiety… and he did manage to decrease the number of panic attacks and also to lift, to experience the panic attacks in a much less distracting way. And he was really pleased, in fact he said he didn't go to therapy afterwards because he felt he was able to… his [actual] words were 'You know, you helped me and now I feel I can deal with that…' So that was quite nice.*"

Male GP, London

"*The other patient I used it on was to do with drug compliance. He's a diabetic and it's actually really poorly controlled. So I… tried to use it on him as well and that's been quite useful because… by discovering why he's not taking the medication and his views about diabetes and the complications etc., I've managed to actually instil some ideas into him as to why he should try and comply with the medication, so I mean it's helped a little bit actually.*"

Chapter 2

Adapting CBT for general practice

- The 'cognitive-behavioural model' (CBM) offers a simple way for GPs to incorporate elements of CBT into 10-minute consultations

- The CBM provides a framework for understanding individual problems in terms of CBT theory

- The approach is relevant to a wide variety of emotional problems including depression, anxiety and psychological difficulties associated with chronic physical disease.

- Developing skills in using the CBM can save time or help use it more effectively

The 'cognitive-behavioural model'

The 'cognitive-behavioural model' (CBM) (*Figure 2.1*) improves the understanding of problems by breaking them down into five areas:

- Thoughts
- Feelings
- Physical reactions/symptoms (biological factors)
- Behaviour
- Environmental factors

The CBM provides an overview or 'map' which enables GPs and patients to understand how these five areas may interact to produce and maintain people's specific problem(s).

The CBM approach was developed to meet the needs of GPs and other health professionals within the primary care setting. This includes taking into account the time limitations of most GP consultations. The CBM can be viewed as another 'tool' to add to the extensive GP 'toolkit' of consulting skills.

Figure 2.1:
Cognitive-behavioural model (CBM) for GP consultations (adapted from Padesky & Mooney, 1990; Williams & Garland, 2002)

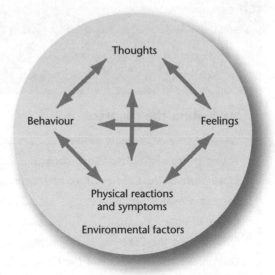

The CBM offers a focused and simple method of incorporating a cognitive-behavioural approach into routine primary care consultations. Whilst the model is derived from the basic theory and principles of CBT (Padesky & Mooney, 1990; Williams & Garland, 2002), it is useful to distinguish the CBM from 'full' or 'standard' CBT, which is carried out in a 'therapy' setting over a longer period of time (see *Box 2.1*).

The CBM also forms a bridge between primary care consultations and mental health services by introducing patients to the theory and approaches of CBT, which can improve the outcome for patients referred onwards for CBT-based interventions.

Box 2.1: Comparison of CBT and the CBM

CBT	CBM
Used in one-hour therapy sessions	Used in routine primary care appointments lasting 10–20 minutes
Used by fully trained CBT practitioners (e.g. therapists, psychologists, nurse practitioners)	Can be used by primary care health professionals (e.g. GPs, practice nurses, health visitors) in routine appointments
Brief intervention: usually involves 6–20 sessions	Continuity of care in general practice often involves fitting CBM approach into long-term relationships with patients
NHS referral usually limited to specific, moderate to severe psychiatric diagnoses and disorders	Useful for a wide range of primary care problems, including mild to moderate difficulties that are fully managed in primary care
Role of CBT practitioner specifically relates to improving psychological problems	Role of GP involves a broad range of responsibilities including management of psychological difficulties, physical disorders, administrative work and achieving specific health care targets
Primary aim of CBT is to teach methods of *making change* in order to alleviate problems and unpleasant symptoms.	Primary aim to enhance *understanding of problems* from a cognitive-behavioural viewpoint. Lack time for use of in-depth cognitive change techniques.
Primary goal to achieve specific patient outcomes	Broader range of useful outcomes. Improving GP–patient relationships and increasing understanding of patients' (and GPs') problems are important goals, in addition to making improvements in patients' symptoms

Taking a 'case formulation' approach

The CBM is derived from the concept of a cognitive-behavioural '*case formulation*'. This is a method for creating a map or overview of individual problems in terms of cognitive-behavioural theory. This provides a framework that enables both patient and therapist to make sense of complex problems, and allows therapy to be tailored to patients' individual needs and problems.

A cognitive-behavioural case formulation provides an overview of a patient's problems in terms of the five areas of the CBM. It includes information about the patient's important beliefs and values and how these may affect their responses to current life events. The formulation also includes any early or significant life experiences, which may have shaped the patient's beliefs about themselves, others and the rest of the world. These 'core beliefs' are discussed in more depth in Chapter 10.

A general model of case formulation is illustrated in *Figure 2.2.*

Figure 2.2:
General model of case formulation

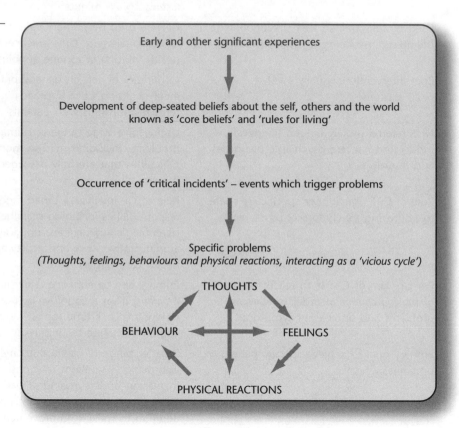

The 'case formulation' approach is central to achieving a good outcome from CBT. There are a number of reasons for this:

1. *Provides clarity and helps to make sense of information*
   A case formulation forms a bridge between cognitive theory and the patient's specific problems. It also provides a structure for the therapy process. This approach enables therapists to work effectively with many different problems, by applying general CBT principles to the specific issues identified by a case formulation.

2. *Improves collaboration and empowers patients*
   Developing and sharing a case formulation helps to build collaborative relationships and actively involves patients in the therapy process.

This teaches patients how to understand and overcome problems themselves – patients learn to become their *own* therapist.

3. *Guiding and directing therapy sessions*
   By providing an accurate understanding of individual patients' problems and their underlying psychological mechanisms, the case formulation helps guide the choice of appropriate treatment strategies.

4. *Therapeutic benefits of the case formulation*
   Developing a case formulation can be therapeutic in its own right. By creating a 'map' or overview of their problems, patients can understand their difficulties better and increase the sense of control over their lives. This encourages patients to believe that change is possible and may help to identify new approaches or solutions to problems.

5. *Overcome difficulties in the CBT process*
   The case formulation can help to understand and predict difficulties in therapy, such as failure to do homework or persistent lateness. These difficulties can be approached as understandable problems for the therapist and patient to address, just like any other issues in the patient's life. This approach can also be applied to any difficulties in the relationship between patient and therapist.

6. *Case formulation for therapists*
   It is often helpful for the therapist to understand themselves and their own reaction to particular patients in terms of their own personal case formulation. For example, if the therapist shares the same, unhelpful belief as the client, it may impede effective therapy. Certain patients may also generate a strong emotional reaction within the therapist. A personal formulation offers a means of understanding and managing this reaction.

From Theory to Practice...	Start using a simple 'case formulation' approach by considering a broad overview of each patient's life. This might mean taking into account the impact of personality, social circumstances and underlying thoughts, beliefs and feelings on any problem.

Reminders: Using a 'case formulation' for CBT

■ General CBT principles are tailored to individual patients using a 'case formulation' – a framework to understand problems in terms of underlying psychological mechanisms

■ Creating a case formulation can help to direct appropriate treatment strategies

■ Using a case formulation to understand and explain problems can be therapeutic in its own right

■ A case formulation can help overcome difficulties in CBT and may also aid a therapist's understanding of their own emotional reactions or difficulties

Making use of the CBM in GP consultations

The CBM approach can be used flexibly depending on the individual needs of both GPs and patients. It can be used in combination with other interventions including medication (for example, antidepressants), counselling, 'bibliotherapy' (using self-help books or leaflets), computerized CBT or as a prelude to CBT itself. Often, the very process of exploring patients' problems using the CBM will help with future management choices.

The principal aim of using the CBM in primary care settings is to help the patient to understand themselves and their problems in greater depth. Other aims of using the CBM are summarized in *Box 2.2*.

Box 2.2: Aims of using the CBM in GP consultations

- To help patients and GPs to understand key problems from a cognitive-behavioural perspective
- To build a collaborative relationship between GP and patient, which encourages patients to take responsibility for their own problems
- To help the patient, where possible, move towards new perspectives and solutions to problems
- To make effective use of the limited time within a GP consultation and maintain realistic goals and expectations of the process by both GP and patient
- To improve diagnosis and to help identify the most appropriate future treatment strategies for individual patients

What are we not trying to achieve?

Identifying what we are *not* trying to achieve when using the CBM in primary care consultations can alleviate some of the pressure that GPs may feel when learning new techniques or attempting to help patients with complex emotional problems.

The GP is *not* trying:

- To change the patient's mind or to persuade them around to the GP's own way of thinking
- To take on extra responsibility for solving a patient's problems
- To become a 'mini' cognitive therapist who can 'cure' patients in 10 minutes
- To use the CBM with every patient in every consultation

Keeping a realistic attitude

Learning to understand patients using the CBM can be a fascinating process which increases the enjoyment and satisfaction taken from consultations. It is helpful to adopt an attitude of 'expectant interest' and to enjoy the '*journey of discovery*' of learning more about a patient, rather than feeling pressurized into providing solutions to the patient's complex problems. In fact, this pressure often arises from a GP's high expectations *of themselves*, rather than coming directly from patients.

It is important to maintain realistic expectations about potential benefits from using the CBM approach. It is *not* possible to carry out 'standard' CBT within 10-minute consultations, but small improvements are often both possible and worthwhile. While this may seem obvious, many GPs have high expectations and may feel disheartened when patients do not improve as much or as quickly as they might wish.

Remember that it may take *time* for patients to fully understand the complex, new information and approach to their problems provided by the CBM. Change may therefore not be immediately apparent within the confines of a 10-minute GP consultation. However, this does not necessarily mean that the process has not been helpful. Allowing the patient space to think about their problems *over time* can often be very effective and useful.

Rather than expecting to identify the 'answer' within the consultation itself, it can be more helpful to harness the time *in between consultations* to make progress. Ending a consultation in an open way, *without* any immediate answers or solutions to problems may encourage patients to spend time reflecting on their difficulties themselves. Patients may leave the consultation with a small spark of new understanding, which develops further and generates change once they have had time to think and assimilate the information into their daily life. This is facilitated by giving the patient a written record of the information gathered to consider in their own time.

Reminders: Keeping a realistic attitude

- Try to remain realistic about potential benefits from using the CBM
- Leaving a consultation 'open' may encourage patients to generate changes in their own lives *over time*
- Pressures to provide rapid solutions for patients often stem from a GP's *own* high expectations and unhelpful beliefs
- It is more helpful to relax and enjoy the 'voyage of discovery' by focusing on understanding patients in more depth

From Theory to Practice...	With one or two patients, try taking an attitude of 'expectant interest' in understanding their problems. Try to reduce the pressure to 'get somewhere' and simply enjoy the 'voyage of discovery' to find out more about the different aspects of their problem(s).
	Remember, that a simple way to change your attitude or beliefs is to change your behaviour. What could you *do* differently to help this process?
	What impact, both positive and negative, does this have on the consultation?

Choice of patients

The CBM is a useful approach for exploring a range of problems including (but not exclusively):

* Depression
* Anxiety and panic attacks
* Phobias including social phobia
* Health anxiety and medically unexplained symptoms
* Low self-esteem
* Obsessive–compulsive disorder
* 'Difficult' or 'heartsink' consultations
* Chronic pain
* Patients with complex social problems
* Psychological elements of chronic disease (including concordance with treatment)
* Promoting healthy lifestyles and behaviours (e.g. smoking cessation, encouraging weight loss)

Should any particular patients be avoided?

As with all consultation techniques, some patients will find the CBM approach more useful than others. However, GPs should try to avoid 'all-or-nothing' views about 'success' or 'failure' of the model with different patients. It is more useful to consider the impact of the CBM on a rating scale, from *'helpful'* to *'unhelpful'*. This should take into account the wide range of potentially useful outcomes for both GP and patient. Remember that the principal aim of the model is to increase *understanding* of the nature of problems rather than to solve them immediately.

Remember that some important, positive outcomes from using the CBM may not be immediately obvious, but may arise later, for example strengthening a relationship with a patient, reducing frequent attendances to surgery in a patient with health anxiety, or facilitating long-term changes in a patient's life.

Box 2.3:
Features suggesting that patients are likely to be suitable for CBT (Safran & Segal, 1990; Wills & Sanders, 1997)

* Able to identify automatic thoughts
* Able to distinguish different emotions
* Accepts responsibility for change
* Understands the rationale for CBT
* Able to develop a good enough relationship with the health professional
* Able to concentrate enough to focus on issues
* The patient's problems are not too severe
* Has some optimism regarding therapy

There are several rating scales which may indicate whether patients are particularly suitable for CBT (*Box 2.3*).

However, this does not mean that cognitive-behavioural approaches should *never* be used in patients who do not display all these features. Standard CBT has been specifically adapted for use with a variety of patients that do not fit these criteria, such as those with chronic depression, personality disorders and even psychoses.

The CBM approach can still be helpful even if patients do not fully fit all of the above criteria. Note that some of these criteria such as 'understanding the rationale for CBT' and 'developing a good enough relationship with the health professional' will be actively promoted and enhanced by effective use of the CBM in consultations.

Nevertheless, especially whilst learning about the CBM, it can be helpful to choose patients who largely fit the criteria for suitability. Later, when you are more familiar with the model, you may feel more confident to use it with a wider variety of patients.

From Theory to Practice	Whilst you are learning about the CBM, it is useful to begin by identifying patients who may be more likely to benefit from the process.
	When you are considering whether to discuss the CBM with patients, try introducing the model subtly by simply asking about their thoughts and feelings.
	Notice that some patients will understand and connect with these concepts more quickly and easily than others.

Factors that may indicate potential difficulties with using the CBM include:

Severe and major psychiatric diagnoses
The CBM is not an alternative for referral to secondary care. Severe cases, such as major depression, should always be fully assessed and referred onwards as appropriate. Using the CBM in a brief consultation may be less appropriate or helpful for these patients.

Strong emotion or affect
Intense feelings during a consultation, such as severe depression or extreme anger, can distort patients' viewpoints and impair their ability to engage and collaborate with the CBM. Reducing such high levels of emotion, for example by defusing anger or reducing anxiety levels, may be important in these cases. The chapters covering individual clinical disorders cover in more detail how to approach this with different problems.

'Heartsink' patients
The CBM is often a very helpful approach to take with some 'heartsink' patients. Nevertheless, for patients with a long history of chronic physical

and/or psychological disorders, it may be unrealistic for GPs to expect major changes from any brief intervention like the CBM. The key is to stay realistic about what can reasonably be achieved. Improving the GP–patient relationship or even working on a GP's own emotional reactions to particular patients may be more important and helpful than trying to change long-standing and ingrained thinking patterns and beliefs in these patients.

Reminders: Choice of patients

- GPs can use the CBM effectively with a wide variety of problems including depression, anxiety and psychological aspects of chronic disease
- The CBM is not a replacement for specialist referral
- The impact of the CBM can be measured in terms of the level of 'helpfulness', which includes a variety of outcomes that are not always immediately apparent
- GPs must maintain realistic expectations about what can be achieved from using the CBM

Incorporating the CBM into consultations

The flexible approach of the CBM enables GPs to use the model in a variety of ways within different practices and patient populations. For example, some GPs choose a particular, pre-booked surgery to practice the techniques. Others may prefer to use simple approaches on a more *ad hoc* basis.

It is often helpful to agree and plan to use the CBM in advance, giving patients time to think about their problems before each appointment. In surgeries where 'double' appointments are a realistic option, some GPs may choose to allocate this time to working through the five areas of the CBM. Other GPs use brief, specific elements of the CBM within a standard 10-minute consultation.

Different areas of the CBM can be discussed during consecutive appointments. This allows the patient time to reflect upon the issues in between consultations. However, the CBM does not have to be viewed as an ongoing commitment for a long period of time. Follow-up can vary from one to several appointments and can be discussed and agreed in advance.

Some different approaches to incorporating the CBM into consultations are shown in *Box 2.4.*

Overcoming barriers to use of the CBM

One of the most useful features of the CBM is that the model itself can be used to help overcome any problems with its use. Turning the CBM 'on itself' is a powerful form of self-examination which can help to make the model useful in a variety of settings.

Box 2.4:
Different approaches to incorporating the CBM into consultations

- Help patients to understand their problems in more depth by breaking down particular issues into the five areas of the CBM
- Take a more focused approach by identifying one or two key areas of the CBM that are particularly important for a patient, such as the interaction between specific thoughts and feelings
- Use the CBM to give coherent explanations of disorders such as anxiety and depression
- Use the CBM as a self-reflective tool after the consultation for understanding GPs' own negative reactions to difficult situations and patients

Box 2.5:
Environmental and organizational factors that may limit use of the CBM

Time constraints/practice organization
- Time pressures – conflict with other clinical/administrative responsibilities
- Appointment systems – lack of pre-booked or double appointments

Patient factors
- Cultural factors, e.g. non-English speaking populations
- Highly complex health needs
- Severe psychiatric conditions or multiple, long-standing complaints
- Willingness to actively participate, including follow-up

Working patterns
- Lack of continuity (e.g. working in a short-term/locum position, part-time workers)
- Variations in GP roles within practice

Wider organizational factors
- Pressure to meet external targets/performance indicators – competing demands on time

Certain environmental and practice organizational factors will inevitably limit how often GPs can use CBM approaches in primary care (see *Box 2.5*). Some factors, such as specific patient characteristics, may be fixed and unchangeable. However, by using the CBM flexibly, according to the particular needs of each GP and practice population, most GPs *are* able to effectively incorporate CBM approaches within their routine practice.

Whilst many organizational factors are genuine barriers to using CBM approaches, certain unhelpful GP beliefs may also be present, which act to compound, rather than solve the problem. It can also often be helpful to use the CBM to evaluate and re-frame these beliefs. This approach is explored in the following case examples.

Time pressures

> ### Case example 2.1: Managing time pressures
>
> Dr K works in a busy surgery in an inner city location. She constantly needs to juggle the conflicting pressures of seeing patients, administrative work and doing home visits. She would like to learn to use CBM strategies as she thinks they might help her and her patients. However, she is very concerned about how much time it will take.
>
> "*I don't have time to use CBT. I am so busy in surgery and I already overrun quite frequently. I just couldn't cope if surgeries became any longer.*"

The statement "*I don't have time to use CBT*" is a 'black-and-white' statement implying that applying a cognitive-behavioural approach will *always* increase time pressures. It may reflect an unrealistic expectation of how much ground 'should' be covered in any given appointment. It may also overestimate how often the approach 'should' be used, perhaps by using it in nearly every consultation, or not at all.

It is more helpful to take a 'shades of grey' approach: implementing cognitive-behavioural techniques can be carried out in small 'chunks' that are manageable and fit within routine appointments. The aim is to make small incremental changes *over time*. It may be surprising to discover how much useful and interesting ground can be covered during a 10-minute consultation.

In fact, cognitive-behavioural approaches to consulting may help GPs use time *more effectively*. Key consultation skills that help to manage time pressures include:

* Setting an agenda
* Writing down key information
* Taking a focused approach
* Listening actively
* Using homework tasks to encourage the patient to utilize time in between appointments to continue progress
* Keeping a realistic attitude about what can be achieved during a 10-minute appointment

The CBM may also help GPs care more effectively for many patients who *already* regularly attend surgeries for support and counselling with emotional difficulties. Investing some time in understanding patients using the CBM may *save* time in the long-term, by allowing more succinct discussions in future consultations or by using the CBM to help understand and manage the consulting behaviour of frequently attending patients.

Like Dr K above, many GPs *already* run late with surgeries and fear that learning CBM techniques will lengthen surgeries and increase pressure upon the

GP. If you do regularly overrun, it can be helpful to use the CBM to reflect upon why this is the case. Environmental factors such as interruptions or short appointment times may be to blame. However, persistent lateness may also relate to certain internal GP factors, such as anxiety about decision-making or difficulty coping with uncertainty. Some GPs hold beliefs such as "It is rude to interrupt patients," which may make it difficult to cope with talkative patients or to bring consultations to a close. Using the CBM to address some of these internal issues may actually alleviate time pressures.

Overall, general practice is a balance between competing pressures, ranging from seeing patients, to meeting clinical targets, to a GP's own self-care. Nevertheless, many GPs chose this career path because of their genuine interest in working with patients, hearing their stories and knowing them as individual people. This aspect of general practice is one of the most interesting and rewarding and is a key feature of the CBM approach. Finding time to maintain interest and enthusiasm in general practice is important to avoid problems such as stress and burnout.

Dr K's unhelpful beliefs could be 'reframed' to take into account the following, alternative perspectives:

> "*I have limited time so I will start by trying to use the CBM in one or two consultations during surgeries that are usually less rushed.*"

> "*I am not trying to achieve miracles – just using small elements of the CBM can still be very helpful within my routine consultations.*"

Reminders: Managing time pressures

- A surprising amount of useful and interesting ground can be covered during a 10-minute consultation
- The approach can be applied in small, manageable 'chunks'
- Using the CBM can save time or help use it more effectively
- The CBM may help GPs understand and overcome problems such as regularly running late in surgeries

---

GP confidence

Case example 2.2: Lack of GP confidence

Dr H is a GP registrar. She does not feel confident in managing patients with mental health problems and other emotional difficulties. She has read about CBT and would like to be able to use it in her consultations. However, she is concerned about trying the techniques with patients.

"*I am not enough of a mental health expert to use CBT in my consultations. I don't want to try as I might fail and look like a fool in front of the patient. I will try it once I am better skilled with these kinds of patient.*"

It is not necessary to be an expert cognitive therapist to use the CBM. Most GPs are *already* highly skilled communicators who balance a wide variety of competing issues within a very short period of time. The CBM encourages GPs to use these existing skills and to build upon them.

Learning any new skill takes time and effort. No one can become an expert without plenty of practice. This can be likened to learning to drive. How realistic would it be to expect to pass your driving test without ever having had any lessons? When learning to drive it is essential to practice so that skills become ingrained.

When learning new knowledge or skills, it is often necessary to alter behaviour (trying out new techniques) before you are able to change thoughts (consolidation of new CBT knowledge and skills) or feelings (increased confidence and reduced anxiety).

So how do we practice and refine our skills in using the CBM? One option is to practice in a safe environment. Using the CBM on yourself or with colleagues to understand your reactions to certain consultations or personal situations can be a very helpful starting point to develop your understanding of the CBM. Another possibility is to attend practical training workshops, which enable participants to practice skills before trying them on patients.

It can be less overwhelming to attempt to introduce individual CBM skills one at a time. For example, you could begin by looking for thoughts and unhelpful thinking styles. Then start to link these to feelings and behaviour. Each chapter of this book includes simple suggestions for turning CBT theory into practice.

GPs may also harbour perfectionist beliefs that they should be able to learn and use the CBM absolutely perfectly straight away. Again, this can be compared to learning to drive. How many novice drivers are able to jump straight into a car and drive perfectly? Making mistakes and overcoming difficulties is a key part of the learning process. Some GPs feel most comfortable if they openly admit to patients that they are learning a new technique and asking whether the patient would be interested in learning about it too. Other GPs simply try out the skills without over-emphasizing the importance or meaning to themselves or the patient. It is helpful to aim to become 'good enough' rather than 'perfect' at using CBM techniques.

A more helpful perspective for Dr H might be:

> "*No one can be perfect at any new skill straight away – I would like to become more confident at using the CBM so it is important to practice.*"
>
> "*I will start by using it on myself….*"
>
> "*I will pick out one or two new things to try each week….*"

Maintaining boundaries – fears of patient dependence

Case example 2.3: Dependency

Dr Y is one of four partners in a medium-sized practice in a busy market town. He has a number of patients who he feels might benefit from CBM approaches. However, he is concerned that these patients may become 'dependent' on him to solve their problems.

"I would like to help these people but I don't want them to become too dependent on me. I am not a therapist. I don't want patients to think they have to come and see me for every single problem. I just don't have time for that."

Concerns about developing patient dependence may relate to unrealistic expectations held by GPs themselves about using the model to solve patients' problems. To encourage patients to take responsibility for their own problems, it is often more helpful for GPs to take a more supportive role in *partnership* with patients. Many of the CBM skills actively promote collaborative working relationships that empower patients to take control of their own problems and lives.

The anxiety relating to possible dependency by patients may also relate to a GP's own beliefs about relationships with patients. It might indicate that the GP lacks confidence or skills in managing patients with excessive or unrealistic demands. In this case, using the CBM to identify any unhelpful beliefs that may impede a GP's assertiveness with certain patients may also be useful.

A more helpful perspective for Dr Y may be:

> *"Hopefully, learning about the CBM will help me to develop collaborative relationships where patients are actually less dependent on me."*

> *"I will focus on building skills to encourage patients to take responsibility for their own problems."*

> *"Perhaps I could also use the CBM to help me cope with demanding patients."*

Reminders: Overcoming barriers to using the CBM

- The CBM can be applied flexibly to help overcome specific environmental difficulties
- It may be important for GPs identify and challenge any unhelpful beliefs that interfere with learning or using the model in practice
- GPs can build confidence in using the approach by learning and practicing the model in stages
- Using cognitive-behavioural approaches can decrease patient dependency on health care professionals

---

From Theory to Practice...	What are the greatest barriers that might prevent you from beginning to use the CBM in your practice?
	Use the CBM to examine these barriers.
	Are there any ways to overcome or alter external factors (e.g. by reducing interruptions or setting aside a specific surgery to practice the technique)?
	Do you hold any beliefs which may be unhelpful in learning about the CBM? Can you think of any ways to challenge or 'reframe' these beliefs?

Chapter 3

Basic principles of CBT

- How people *think* affects how they *feel* (emotionally and physically) and how they *behave*

- People's reactions to particular situations are individual and unique

- Negative thoughts, feelings, physical symptoms and behaviour often link to form 'vicious cycles'

- Identifying and breaking vicious cycles is a key element of the CBT process

The relationship between thoughts, feelings and behaviour

The fundamental principle of CBT is that the way people *think* in a specific situation will affect how they *feel* emotionally and physically, and also alters their *behaviour*.

In depression and anxiety, people tend to think in more extreme and unhelpful ways. They may focus on negative self-concepts, such as viewing themselves as worthless, a failure or vulnerable to danger. Behaviour also alters, perhaps by reducing activity or avoiding certain situations. People may develop new unhelpful behaviours such as excessive drinking, self-harming or repeated reassurance-seeking. This exacerbates emotional distress in the form of a vicious cycle.

CBT teaches patients to identify unhelpful patterns of thinking and behaviour and to develop new, more helpful thoughts and reactions. Of course, CBT is not trying to eliminate emotional responses altogether! Appropriate emotion is a normal, healthy and necessary response to life's changing situations. However, certain responses, particularly if repetitive, may start to form unhelpful, negative patterns. The key is to identify how thoughts, feelings and behaviours are interacting in any one individual at any time in order to make informed choices about helpful ways to move forwards.

Using a cognitive-behavioural approach, problems can be broken down into the five areas of the CBM: thoughts, feelings, physical symptoms, behaviour and environmental factors/triggers (*Figure 2.1*)

Different perspectives for the same situation

It is important to separate people's *internal reactions* from the *external situations* that have triggered a particular response. Whilst people commonly assume that "anyone would feel the same as me in this situation," in reality, a wide variety of individual reactions can occur in response to the same situation.

3.1 Consider the following situation:	You have cooked dinner for a friend, who is usually very reliable. An hour after she was due to arrive, there is still no sign and you have received no phone call...

How would you react in this situation? The following table illustrates four different possible reactions, broken down into thoughts with their corresponding feelings and behaviours:

Event	A friend is an hour late for dinner…			
Thought	*"How dare she do this to me! She is so inconsiderate and rude!"*	*"She probably didn't want to come because she doesn't really like me. I'm such a loser."*	*"What if she's had an accident? She could be seriously hurt."*	*"I expect she's stuck in traffic. At least I have extra time to prepare dinner."*
Feelings	Anger	Depression	Anxiety	Relieved
Possible behaviour	Tell her off or be unfriendly when she arrives	Withdraw from people and stop asking them over	Phone local hospitals	Continue preparing dinner

The chart illustrates that how people feel and behave in a particular situation is likely to correspond to their individual thoughts and beliefs. These will vary from person to person. On different occasions, the same individual may also react differently, perhaps depending on their mood or on other circumstances and life events.

Any of these responses may be appropriate in different circumstances. But when people suffer from emotional disorders, they often react negatively to nearly every situation that they encounter. This results in a persistently anxious or depressed mood which is further maintained by unhelpful behaviour patterns as a 'vicious cycle'.

Reflective exercise 3.1: **Different perspectives for the same situation**

As in the previous example, consider the variety of feelings, thoughts and behaviours that different individuals may experience in the following situations:

- A friend walks past on the street and ignores you
- Missing out on a promotion
- Disaster victims reacting in different ways

From Theory to Practice… Start becoming aware of the diverse range of reactions both in yourself and others to different situations in everyday life. Take particular note of the following:

- Are there links betweens people's thoughts, feelings and how they behave?
- What is the impact of this behaviour? How is it helpful or unhelpful?

Understanding thoughts and cognitions

What are thoughts?

'Thoughts' are words and visual images that pass through people's minds. The term encompasses a variety of mental processes including attitudes, ideas, expectations, memories, beliefs and images. The evaluation of thoughts and thinking styles comprises the 'cognitive' element of CBT.

As implied by the term, *automatic* thoughts are instantaneous, unplanned thoughts which flow through our minds throughout the day in response to events. 'Negative automatic thoughts', which assume the worst in any given situation, are common in disorders such as depression and anxiety.

Automatic thoughts often *seem* plausible although they are not necessarily accurate or realistic. In the example above, the person whose friend is late for dinner does not actually know the real reason for this event. But although negative automatic thoughts are merely guesses or assumptions, they still have *consequences* by altering people's feelings and subsequent behaviour.

Remember that thoughts can take the form of both words and images. For example, a woman who is terrified of driving may experience verbal fears such as "*I might crash and die if I get in the car.*" She may also experience intense, evocative images such as an image of her own dead body in the mangled remains of a crashed car on the motorway. Clearly, such images will have a powerful influence on her feelings.

Automatic thoughts often arise very rapidly and may be difficult to catch in a particular situation. They are conscious processes but they may occur outside the focus of immediate awareness. However, with practice, most people can learn to identify key automatic thoughts, such as those associated with powerful emotions.

Chains of thoughts

Thoughts rarely occur individually – one thought about a particular issue commonly leads to others in a 'cascade'. People often experience an 'explosion' of thoughts occurring in rapid succession.

Let's reconsider the previous example of different ways to view the same situation. Imagine that Sally, a 25-year old student, is waiting for her friend to arrive for dinner. She feels sad and depressed because she has begun to think that her friend does not really like her. She may have a sequence of thoughts such as:

⇒ My friend is late for dinner

⇒ She must have forgotten about the invitation

⇒ She probably had something more interesting or important to do

⇒ This must mean that she thinks I am boring

⇒ She probably doesn't really like me

⇒ No one seems to really care about me or make any effort for me

⇒ What's wrong with me?

⇒ No one ever likes me

⇒ There is no point in inviting anyone to visit me – they won't want to come

⇒ It must be because I am a really horrible, boring person

⇒ My life is meaningless and empty

Such a cascade is often very rapid – occurring within a few seconds – and Sally may not be consciously aware of all of the steps. However, rather than simply feeling a little disappointed or put out that her friend has not yet arrived, she begins to feel very depressed and low because the cascade of thoughts has led to the conclusion that she is boring and her life is meaningless.

The process of CBT teaches patients to view their thoughts as merely *hypotheses* or *guesses* to be tested against reality, rather than absolute fact. It may not be possible to alter the immediate, automatic thought that occurs in response to a particular event. However, patients *can* learn to identify and test out whether their automatic thoughts represent a realistic assess-ment of the situation or whether another perspective may be more accurate and helpful. This process of identifying a more balanced perspective may also reduce negative feelings.

From Theory to Practice...	When people become distressed, take time to try to understand the underlying cascades of thoughts that may be present. You could try this out in one or two clinics. Make an effort to listen carefully and gently ask questions such as: *"What was going through your mind...?"* *"What is it about this situation that really upsets you?"*

Reminders: Understanding thoughts

■ 'Thoughts' are a variety of processes including words, memories and images

■ 'Negative automatic thoughts' occur spontaneously in response to daily events. They may not be realistic but can still worsen mood and alter behaviour

■ CBT aims to help patients to view thoughts as *theories* or *guesses*

■ Altering negative thoughts can improve the way people feel

Making sense of feelings

In CBT terminology, 'feelings' are viewed as emotions or moods, such as feeling happy, excited, angry, sad, frustrated, embarrassed or fearful. Many of these can be categorized into groups. Some of the common *negative* feelings include the following:

- **Sadness and loss:** e.g. feeling low, down, unhappy, depressed, miserable, sad, fed up, disappointed
- **Guilt and shame:** e.g. ashamed, guilty, embarrassed, humiliated, mortified
- **Anxiety and fear:** e.g. feeling nervous, tense, frightened, anxious, worried, afraid, scared, panicky, terrified, petrified
- **Anger and hurt:** e.g. feeling annoyed, irritated, frustrated, cross, exasperated, angry, furious, mad, livid, infuriated, hurt

People use a variety of words to describe feelings. For example, a patient may describe feeling 'upset.' This might represent feelings of sadness, hurt, anger or even guilt. It can be very important to clarify what an individual patient actually means, using questions such as:

> *"What did feeling 'upset' mean for you in this situation? Are there any other ways to describe how you felt so that I can fully understand what you mean?"*

Patients may have difficulty in accurately identifying feelings. Some, particularly men, may view feelings and emotions as a sign of 'weakness'. Others may be experiencing such powerful emotions that they have developed a coping strategy of ignoring or denying that these feelings exist. In these cases, patients can be slowly encouraged to identify and monitor different feelings.

Rating feelings

It is often helpful for patients to learn to rate the intensity of their feelings, on a scale from 0 to 100, using a visual rating scale for this (*Figure 3.1*):

Figure 3.1: Rating scale for intensity of feelings (adapted from Greenberger & Padesky, 1995a)

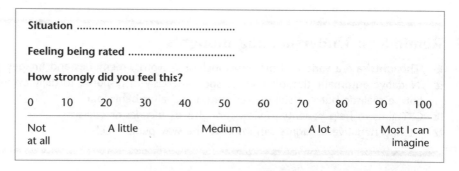

| Situation .... |
| Feeling being rated .... |
| How strongly did you feel this? |

| 0 | 10 | 20 | 30 | 40 | 50 | 60 | 70 | 80 | 90 | 100 |

| Not at all | | A little | | | Medium | | | A lot | | Most I can imagine |

Monitoring the intensity of feelings usually shows that feelings fluctuate widely over a period of time. This can be helpful in conditions such as depression, where patients may overlook or discount positive experiences and hold beliefs such as:

"I always feel terrible."

"I never enjoy anything – I'm constantly depressed and anxious."

Identifying even minor fluctuations in mood begins to challenge the depressed person's view that life is *completely terrible*. It opens up the possibility that there may be some, small positive things in life *already* and that the patient's task is to build upon these. This can offer hope and encouragement to patients and make the task of overcoming depression seem less overwhelming.

It is also useful to identify and record any changes in intensity of feelings when the patient tries a new strategy to cope with their difficulties. For example, a depressed person could record how they feel before and after going for a walk. This helps reinforce the benefit of particular behaviours and offers objective measure of the patient's progress. Even a small reduction in negative feelings, perhaps from 80 down to 60, still represents an important improvement in mood.

Reminders: Making sense of feelings

■ Learning to identify feelings helps patients understand their experiences
■ People use a variety of words to describe feelings so it is important to clarify exactly what they mean
■ Monitoring fluctuations in the intensity of feelings helps monitor improvement in CBT

From Theory to Practice...	When patients are emotionally upset, make a particular effort to identify which feelings are the strongest and the most distressing
	Ask patients to rate how the intensity of feelings are on a scale from 0 to 100
	Do these feelings fluctuate over time? What is the impact of particular helpful/unhelpful behaviour on the intensity of feelings?

The relationship between thoughts and feelings

Separating thoughts from feelings

Separating thoughts and feelings can make complex emotional reactions seem more understandable. As a general rule, feelings and moods can usually be described in one descriptive word (e.g. anger, sadness, fear). If it takes more than one word to describe a mood, this is likely to be describing a *thought* rather than a *feeling*.

Differentiating between thoughts and feelings is central to using a cognitive-behavioural approach. Remember that it is nearly always unhelpful to challenge or question the validity of a patient's feelings. These are subjective experiences that can only be felt and described by that individual. However, it may be possible to re-frame any associated unhelpful thoughts and beliefs. This often helps to alter negative feelings indirectly.

In the English language, it is common to insert the word 'feel' into a statement which is actually a thought. It is usually used to indicate that the speaker is aware that the thought or belief is their own opinion. It is not usually helpful to overtly correct any patient's 'mistakes' if they confuse thoughts and feelings. This can seem patronizing and may damage your relationship with them. It is often more useful to simply lead by example. Reflect back the patient's words and ask for any associated emotions. Be prepared to ask several times if the patient does not understand your meaning.

For example, a patient may say:

"I feel that my husband is really upset with me."

This statement is a thought not a feeling. In order to elicit the feeling, you could ask:

"How does it make you feel when you think that your husband is upset with you?"

The patient may reply:

"I feel that he is starting to drift away from me and that he might want to leave me."

Again, this is another thought. You could react to this by asking again:

"And how do you feel about the idea that your husband may be drifting away from you and might want to leave you?"

The patient may then respond by describing her feelings about the situation:

"I feel really anxious and terrified. I don't know how I would cope on my own."

Connections between thoughts and feelings

There is usually a logical relationship between the thoughts and feelings expressed by patients. For example, a patient thinking *"My life is a total disaster and I am a failure as a person,"* is likely to feel depressed and low. Similarly, anxious people tend to worry about the potential dangers everywhere and angry people think about the ways they have been hurt or wronged.

This can help health professionals to develop genuine empathy for the patient's experience. It becomes possible to put ourselves into the patient's shoes by imagining: "If I thought like that then I would also expect to feel…"

Reflective **Linking thoughts and feelings**

exercise In the following exercise, cover the right hand column and consider which
3.2: feelings you might expect to coincide with the following list of thoughts:

Thought	Possible feeling(s)
"What if I give a terrible speech to my colleagues? It might go down like a lead balloon and they will think I'm incompetent."	Anxiety Fear
"I'm worthless. No one wants me."	Depression Sadness
"My son failed to get to university. It's all my fault. I'm a bad parent."	Guilt
"I showed myself up in public by swearing at those people."	Shame
"I always do my best for him. Why doesn't he do his best for me?"	Hurt
"He shouldn't interrupt me. He's a thoughtless idiot."	Anger

There is a reciprocal relationship between thoughts and feelings. In other words, thinking negatively is likely to make people feel bad and feeling low will also make people think more negatively. The more intensely we experience a particular emotion, the more extreme the associated thinking is likely to be.

This two-way relationship between thoughts and feelings may be something of a 'chicken and egg' situation. Fortunately, it is not really necessary for effective CBT to determine which came first. Instead, we focus on identifying the relevant thoughts and feelings. This helps the patient discover ways of breaking the negative cycle and feeling better.

Reminders: Relationships between thoughts and feelings

■ Separating thoughts and feelings can make complex emotional reactions seem more understandable
■ Trying to understand the logical relationship between particular thoughts and feelings helps GPs develop empathy for a patient's experiences
■ Altering the negative thoughts and behaviours that underlie negative feelings can improve mood

Making sense of complex situations

Learning to distinguish between thoughts, feelings, behaviours and situations is an important skill. When discussing problems, patients often present huge amounts of information as a jumbled mix of thoughts, feelings and events. Taking time to break these down into the five areas of the CBM (situation/events, thoughts, feelings, physical symptoms) can give both GP and patient a sense of order and control over the problem.

Case example 3.1: Using the CBM to make sense of complex situations

---

Jane is a 30-year old single parent. In the following dialogue, she discusses some of her concerns about her 10-year old son Adam, who is having difficulty at school. Jane is struggling to juggle working full-time alongside bringing up her son, and feels increasingly depressed and low.

GP Can you tell me what has been going on with Adam that has been getting you down recently?

Jane Well, he has been really misbehaving at school lately. I got called in to see his teacher last week. He was doing so well last year, and now he doesn't concentrate and is near the bottom of the class.

GP I see. That must be quite a worry for you.

Jane Oh yes, it is. He is being really cheeky at home too. I don't know what will happen to him. And what with work being so busy right now, I'm just at the end of my tether. It makes me feel so low I just I don't think I can cope any more. Honestly, I'm so tired and fed up with it all. Everything is just a complete mess. When I went to see his teacher, I'm sure she blamed me for everything.

GP What makes you say that?

Jane Well, to start with, I was 15 minutes late to see her because I got held up at work. She must have thought that I am a terrible mother. And then she asked if there were any problems at home. I didn't know what to say. But later on I started thinking about it. Maybe she's right, I *am* a bad mother. I've been too busy at work to give him the time he needs. I've failed and now his school work is suffering. I feel so useless. [*Looks very tearful*]

continued

Jane's problems can be broken down into:

Situation/events   Adam misbehaving at school and at home
                        Adam's performance at school going downhill
                        Work is busy
                        Being called in to see Adam's teacher

Thoughts   *"I'm at the end of my tether."*
                        "I don't think I can cope any more."
                        "Everything is a complete mess."
                        "Adam's teacher blames me for it all" – she thinks I'm a
                        terrible mother.
                        "I am a bad mother."
                        "I've failed."
                        "I'm useless."

Feelings   Low
                        Fed up

Physical symptoms   Tired

Breaking the problem down in this way enables Jane to separate the problems with Adam and his school work from her own thoughts of inadequacy and feelings of low mood. Although related, these issues are *separate* and should be considered independently.

Problem-solving techniques may help to resolve some of the complex difficulties she is facing in her life, such as coping as a single mother with a busy job. However, it is also important to look at some of her negative thinking styles and behaviours which may be adding to her problems rather than solving them.

From Theory to Practice...	Try breaking down a simple problem into different areas: Situation, Thoughts, Feelings, Behaviour and Physical reactions.

Unhelpful thinking styles

Many negative thoughts represent an unhelpful way of looking at the world, which simply worsens problems. Such thoughts often fall into characteristic patterns known as *unhelpful thinking styles* (*Box 3.1*). These are distorted or skewed ways of viewing the world.

Notice that these patterns are described as 'unhelpful' rather than 'wrong'. Otherwise, some patients may begin to blame themselves for thinking in a 'bad' way and may actually feel worse. For example, a depressed person may think: "*Even my thinking is wrong. It is all my fault that I am depressed. I am a complete failure...*" Of course, this statement itself contains several examples of unhelpful thinking styles! It can also be helpful to remind patients that unhelpful thinking styles are common and everyone uses them sometimes. Nevertheless, looking for an alternative view may help people to feel better.

Identifying these unhelpful or distorted thinking patterns provides the first step towards balanced thinking and improved moods. This can be very useful in reducing negative emotion and in finding solutions to seemingly impossible problems. It can be helpful to give patients some written information about negative thinking styles.

Box 3.1: Unhelpful thinking styles

Unhelpful thinking style	Alternative perspective
All or nothing ('black-and-white') thinking	**See things as 'shades of grey'**
You view events or people in 'all or nothing' terms, which is hardly ever accurate: *"Nobody likes me."* *"Anything less than complete perfection means total failure."*	It is rare for anything to ever be either 100% perfect or a complete disaster. Try to be realistic and take into account both positive and negative events.
Negative view of yourself	**Be fair to yourself**
You are very self-critical and negative about yourself: *"I always mess things up."* *"I am a complete idiot for making that mistake."* Being tougher on yourself than others is unfair and can make you feel bad.	Don't forget about all your achievements in life, both small and large. It is impossible for anyone to mess absolutely *everything* up! Would you be as critical if it was your best friend? What would you say to them in the same situation? It is only fair to use the same rules for ourselves as for others!
Mind reading (negative view about how others see you)	**Don't jump to the worst conclusion!**
You tend to assume that others think badly of you: *"He thinks I'm a loser."* *"She must think I'm such an idiot."* You might also give too much importance to someone else's opinion: *"Because he didn't like me it must mean I'm a really boring person."*	Try not to assume the worst about what others think about you – it may not really be true. Others are often more concerned with their own problems than what you have said or done. Even if one person did think something negative, does that really matter so much? Nobody can be liked by everybody at all times. Keep in mind the opinions of the people who like and care about you.
Catastrophic thinking	**Keep a realistic view of the future**
You expect things to go badly and assume that the worst will happen: *"I'll never get that job."* *"I'm not going out tonight, I won't enjoy it at all."*	No one can really be certain what will happen in the future: it is usually a mixture of good and bad things. Try to be realistic. Things may not be perfect but they may be OK.

continued

Assuming the worst will make you feel bad and can make you give up before you even start.	Remember, if you don't try, you won't get anywhere! Keep trying and see what happens.
'What if...?" statements	**Be realistic and focus on solutions**
You constantly worry about future problems and disasters but forget to focus on planning ways to cope with these difficulties: "What if I get anxious when I go to the shops?" "What I don't get the job?" "What if he thinks I'm stupid?"	The worst may not happen! And, don't forget that you could probably cope even if things did go wrong! You have undoubtedly survived plenty of difficult situations in the past. Focus on how you can *cope* with difficulties rather than continually thinking about potential disasters. Write your solutions down on paper.
Blaming yourself (taking too much responsibility for problems)	**Share the responsibility fairly**
You feel a lot of pressure for things to go . well, and blame yourself for any problems, even if these things are outside your control You may forget that some events are also caused by other people. "It is my fault that my partner cheated on me." "I'm a bad mother because my son failed his exams."	Remember that you are not the only person who is responsible for problems. Make a list of *all* the people who are involved or have some responsibility for the situation you are worried about. Put yourself on the list at the end. You might discover that, although you do have some responsibility, *it is not entirely your fault.*
'Should' statements	**Switch "should" to "would prefer to..."**
You focus on how *you* believe things *should* be, rather than how they really are. This can make you feel frustrated and fed up, and gets in the way of solving the problem: "I should never make any mistakes"	Try to avoid blanket rules like "I should always..." which are usually extreme and unrealistic. Remember that making mistakes or facing difficult situations is sometimes inevitable. Focus on what you can do to improve things. "I would like to avoid mistakes if possible, but no one can be perfect."
Blaming others	**Stop blaming and focus on solving problems**
You focus on others as the source of your negative feelings. Blaming others can make you feel frustrated and out of control – after all you do not have the power to change other people! Blaming others may make you angry and stop you seeing ways to help yourself "She's to blame for the way I feel so low." "He made me get angry."	Remember that how we feel depends on how we view a particular situation – so ultimately we are responsible for our own feelings. It may be more helpful to accept that life and other people are never perfect. Feeling angry doesn't make things any better! Instead of focusing on others' faults, (which you cannot change), focus on your own needs and how you could make things better *for yourself.*

Case example 3.2: Identifying unhelpful thinking styles

Take another look at the dialogue between Jane and her GP on page 34 What unhelpful thinking styles can be identified there? Notice that more than one unhelpful thinking style may be present within the same statement.

Thoughts	Unhelpful thinking style(s)
"Everything is a complete mess."	All or nothing thinking
"Adam's teacher blames me for it all."	Mind-reading
"I'm a bad mother."	Blaming yourself
	Negative view of yourself
"I've failed."	All or nothing thinking
	Negative view of yourself
"I don't think I can cope any more."	Negative view of the future
"I'm useless."	All or nothing thinking
	Negative view of yourself

Once these negative thoughts and unhelpful thinking styles have been identified, the patient may be able to find a new way to look at the situation. For example, Jane's thought *"Everything is a complete mess,"* could be replaced with *"Things are difficult but not everything is a mess. Things could certainly be worse! We have a nice home and Adam is healthy and well."*

In Chapter 6, we will look in more detail at how to change thoughts or unhelpful thinking styles.

From Theory to Practice...	Keep an eye out for unhelpful thinking styles. You may notice how common they are in everyday conversation and on TV.
	It is often worth familiarizing yourself with two or three particularly common unhelpful thinking styles.
	Which unhelpful styles do you notice most often? Which do you think have the biggest impact on people?

CBT and positive thinking

CBT is *not* simply about thinking positively. Overly positive thinking has the same problem as excessively negative thinking: it is often inaccurate and unhelpful. For example, if a patient keeps telling herself to "Think positively – everything is fine," there is a risk that her problems may actually get worse because she is not doing anything useful to solve them.

CBT encourages *realistic* thinking. This means taking into account both positive and negative aspects of any problem. Hopefully, by taking this broad perspective, people better equipped to deal with the issues that they face in life.

Reminders: Unhelpful thinking styles

■ 'Unhelpful thinking styles' are distorted ways of looking at the world which are unrealistic and worsen problems
■ They are commonly used in everyday language
■ Identifying unhelpful thinking patterns provides the first step towards balanced thinking and improved moods
■ CBT encourages *realistic* rather than simply positive thinking

The role of behaviour

Identifying and changing unhelpful behaviour plays a key part in the CBT process. 'Behaviour' refers to observable actions that people carry out, or what they *do*. Such behaviour can maintain or worsen people's problems in a 'vicious cycle'.

For example, many depressed people become withdrawn and isolated. They may stop going out or stay in bed for long periods. This behaviour

Case example 3.3: The role of behaviour in maintaining problems (I)

John is 25. He is single and works as a computer programmer. He has been suffering from depression for about six months and is feeling increasingly isolated and lonely. He would like to find a girlfriend but he believes that women see him as boring and unattractive, so he lacks the confidence to talk to them.

Trigger   At a work social gathering, he is approached by Elaine, a female colleague who sits near him in the office

Thoughts   *"I am boring and inadequate"*
"No woman would ever find me attractive or interesting"
"Elaine must think I'm a real loser"

Feelings   Low and depressed

Increased belief that he is boring and unattractive:
"No one was interested in talking to me at the party"
Lack of social contact – feels more isolated and lonely
Reduced opportunity to meet potential partners

Behaviour   Makes excuses and abruptly walks away from Elaine
Goes home early
Turns down invitation to the next office party

usually makes people feel much worse. Both the inactivity, which gives more time to ruminate on negative thoughts, and the lack of enjoyable activities in life result in deepened feelings of depression and sadness.

Breaking vicious cycles with behavioural changes

Changing behaviour can be one of the most powerful ways to break negative cycles and improve a patient's symptoms. This is often the easiest point in the cycle to make changes – it is possible to *behave* differently, irrespective of how we think or feel. This is a very powerful strategy for making positive change. Altering behaviour can have a marked impact on all other areas of the CBM, including thoughts, feelings and even physical symptoms.

The patient can be encouraged to behave *'as if'* they feel better or differently rather than waiting to feel less depressed or anxious before making changes in behaviour.

Case example 3.4: The role of behaviour in maintaining problems (II)

Annie is 35 and has suffering from mild depression and low self-esteem for several years. She has an unfulfilling job as a cleaner. She is married with two children who are boisterous and demanding. She has recently been having problems in the relationship with her husband, who she feels does not offer enough support. She does not have many close friends and is feeling increasingly isolated and lonely. Her husband has been out of work for 6 months and Annie fears that he may have developed depression himself, though he refuses to see his GP about it.

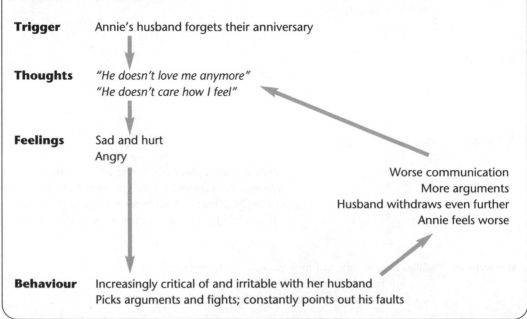

Trigger   Annie's husband forgets their anniversary

Thoughts   *"He doesn't love me anymore"*
                 "He doesn't care how I feel"

Feelings   Sad and hurt
                 Angry

                                              Worse communication
                                                   More arguments
                                      Husband withdraws even further
                                               Annie feels worse

Behaviour   Increasingly critical of and irritable with her husband
                 Picks arguments and fights; constantly points out his faults

Encouraging behavioural change is a particularly useful and effective strategy to use within the time limitations of the primary care setting. We will look in more detail at how to encourage behavioural change in Chapter 8.

Reminders: The role of behaviour

- Unhelpful behaviours can maintain or worsen problems as a vicious cycle
- Altering behaviour is a powerful way to break vicious cycles and make positive change
- Behaving 'as if' you feel differently will improve negative feelings and thoughts
- Encouraging positive changes in behaviour is a very useful strategy for the primary care setting

From Theory to Practice...	In one or two surgeries, focus closely on the impact of behaviour on peoples' experiences: • What kinds of helpful or unhelpful behaviour do you notice? • Does any behaviour result in a vicious cycle which makes problems worse?

Physical reactions and symptoms

Thoughts and feelings can also alter physical and biological reactions. Reading a scary book can lead to a rapid heart rate or sweaty palms as the reader imagines a frightening scene. Thinking about an exciting or enjoyable future event can lead to tingles down the spine or butterflies in the stomach.

In panic disorder, physical reactions play a key role in maintaining the vicious cycle of anxiety. Here, patients misinterpret the meaning of the physical symptoms that they experience. Anxiety and the adrenaline response result in physiological changes such as a raise in heart rate or rapid breathing. The patient notices these changes and mistakenly believes that the symptoms indicate a potentially severe illness, such as a heart attack. This terrifying thought simply increases anxiety as a vicious cycle (*Figure 3.2*).

Changes in physical and biological processes also play an important role in the development and maintenance of depression. Physical symptoms such as lethargy and tiredness often result in negative thoughts and unhelpful behaviour, including excessive resting and reduced enjoyable activities. Biochemical changes, such as reduced serotonin levels in the brain, are also important.

The CBM takes a holistic approach to understanding depression (*Figure 3.3*). This takes into account the role of physical symptoms and biochemical changes as well as other characteristic features of depression, such as negative thinking and unhelpful behaviour. Making positive changes in thoughts and behaviour can therefore be viewed as complementary to 'biological' treatment strategies such as antidepressant medication.

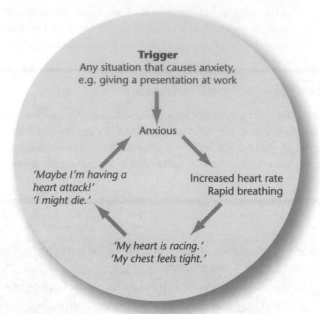

This approach can give patients a greater understanding and sense of control over disorders such as depression. For example, it can encourage patients who view their condition as solely due to changes in their brain biochemistry, to try different approaches in addition to or instead of drug therapy. It can also be helpful in providing a rationale for the use of antidepressants in patients who view their depression as predominantly caused by stressful life events.

In patients with physical disorders, physical symptoms are a key area to include within the CBM approach. People react in very different ways to the experience of physical illness. For example, someone who develops a disorder that limits mobility, perhaps arthritis, may have negative thoughts such as: "My life is completely ruined now I am unable to get around like I used to." These thoughts are likely to have a negative impact on mood and the person may respond by isolating themselves from friends and family.

Feeling depressed and low is also likely to worsen physical symptoms such as pain. The role of CBT and the CBM in these cases is to help facilitate adjustment to and coping with the disorder. This may even improve physical symptoms themselves by breaking vicious cycles of thoughts, feelings and behaviours that may be worsening the problem (see Chapter 15).

Reminders: The role of physical reactions and symptoms

■ Different thoughts and feelings will affect physical reactions of the body
■ Physical symptoms play a key role in maintaining problems such as panic disorder and depression
■ Altering unhelpful thoughts and behaviours can improve mood and help patients cope better with physical disorders and chronic disease

Figure 3.3: CBM of depression

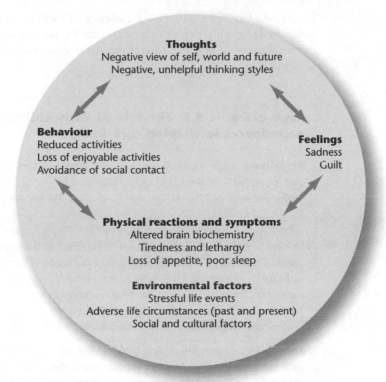

Thoughts
Negative view of self, world and future
Negative, unhelpful thinking styles

Behaviour
Reduced activities
Loss of enjoyable activities
Avoidance of social contact

Feelings
Sadness
Guilt

Physical reactions and symptoms
Altered brain biochemistry
Tiredness and lethargy
Loss of appetite, poor sleep

Environmental factors
Stressful life events
Adverse life circumstances (past and present)
Social and cultural factors

From Theory to Practice...	Start to notice the connections between physical symptoms, thoughts and feelings: • In one or two patients with emotional distress, remember to ask about associated physical changes • In one or two patients presenting with physical symptoms, try to identify what they think and feel about their symptoms or their disorder

The role of environment, social circumstances and culture

A variety of environmental factors may influence people's lives and experiences. This includes early childhood experiences, social and cultural factors.

Early experiences and core beliefs

Early childhood experiences shape people's beliefs about themselves, others and the rest of the world. This can contribute to the formation of deep-rooted beliefs known as 'rules', 'assumptions' and 'core beliefs'. The presence of certain underlying beliefs can help to explain why particular individuals develop depression or anxiety in the face of specific stressful life circumstances or events. More about these types of belief will be covered in Chapter 10.

Case example 3.5: The role of early childhood experiences in shaping core beliefs

Roger grew up in a family environment with a distant and aloof father who was often busy at work. His father was also highly critical of others. Roger's major contact with his father was to discuss the results of his schoolwork. If Roger did badly at school, his father would react angrily saying: "If you fail at school, you will never get anywhere in life." Roger worked harder and harder, hoping to gain his father's approval. He started achieving high grades in most subjects. However, his father would always pick up on any areas where he was not top of the class: "You only came second in maths. You never do well enough…." No matter how hard he worked, his father continued to criticize Roger and comment on his faults. Consequently, Roger developed deep-seated, core beliefs that he was inadequate, a failure and that he was stupid.

Later in life, despite becoming a successful banker, Roger still retained some of these beliefs about himself. He became a perfectionist, believing that "*As long as I am successful in every way then I am OK. But, coming second in anything means total failure.*" These rules drove him to overwork and become highly competitive in everything he did. As long as he remained successful, he felt confident in himself.

However, along with several of his colleagues, Roger was unexpectedly made redundant from work. This life event triggered the reactivation of his negative beliefs about his own failure and stupidity. Given these underlying beliefs, it is unsurprising that Roger found it difficult to cope with the perceived failure of redundancy. In this situation, his reactivated core beliefs resulted in a cascade of negative thoughts and feelings, which gradually developed into depression.

Social and environmental circumstances

The social and environmental circumstances of daily life also play a major role in determining individual people's vulnerability to emotional disorders and distress.

People are much more likely to feel unhappy and low in situations where they feel:

- Unloved or uncared for
- An outsider – not part of any group
- Unsupported or abandoned

- Rejected by others
- Unattractive to self or others
- Unappreciated or not valued by others
- They have low status or experience a loss of status
- A lack of supporting network: friends and family
- A lack of social support, e.g. religious or local community

Socio-economically deprived patients often experience particularly challenging environmental and social circumstances. Nevertheless, emotional disorders are not *inevitable* consequences of financial hardship or other social difficulties. Patients with these problems may still benefit greatly from cognitive-behavioural approaches to their problems. CBT can be an effective approach for people from all walks of life.

Life events

Experiencing a major life event makes individuals more likely to develop an emotional disorder such as depression. Important life events include the death of a close relative or friend, moving house, loss of a job, the break-down of a relationship or the birth of a child. The development of physical illness and disease also increases the risk of depression.

The vulnerability of specific individuals to develop an emotional disorder in response to particular life events will be influenced by several factors including previous life experiences and core beliefs. The degree of 'resilience' that people have developed is also a key factor. This is an ability to cope with or bounce back from difficult situations. Developing resilience can enhance people's ability to cope with adverse life circumstances and events.

Cultural and other social factors

People are also influenced by many other factors including cultural/ethnic backgrounds, religion, family beliefs, gender roles, work environments and the media. These factors, both past and present, influence the way people think and feel about themselves and events in their lives.

Cultural factors play a powerful role in shaping any person's norms and values, and strongly influence their beliefs about themselves and the world. Health professionals must be sensitive to the possibility of different cultural perspectives and norms. It is possible to incorrectly label a patient's own beliefs as 'unhelpful' when these beliefs actually represent a normal cultural perspective for that individual.

If you regularly see patients from a particular cultural group, it can be helpful to educate yourself about that culture in order to better understand the context of these patients' experiences. However, it is also important not to make too many assumptions about the beliefs held by people from particular cultures. Instead, help the individual to evaluate their own beliefs within the context of their own personal and cultural perspective.

Discussing cultural issues with patients can sometimes help them to clarify beliefs and values which they may have held for many years but never articulated. By openly discussing culture with patients – including honestly admitting your knowledge or lack of understanding of a particular culture – and asking for feedback on any cultural assumptions that may be made by the CBM process, you will be able to help the patient to make sense of their problems themselves.

Reminders: Social and environmental factors

■ Important early life experiences influence an individual's beliefs about themselves, others and the world
■ Cultural and social factors have a strong influence on people's values, norms and beliefs
■ Major life events increase the risk of developing emotional disorders
■ Using a CBM approach can enhance people's ability to cope with adverse environmental circumstances

Chapter 4

Working through the stages of the CBM

- Identifying information from all five areas of the CBM helps make sense of problems

- The broad perspective of the CBM can help identify aspects of problems which are important but which have not previously been considered

- Finding relationships between different areas of a problem can help identify new coping strategies or solutions

Introducing the CBM to patients

It is important to give patients a clear rationale for using the CBM approach, as it may be different to anything they have encountered in the past. This also helps to develop a partnership with patients, who must understand the model in order to collaborate and take an active role.

A simple way to introduce the CBM might be to say:

> "*I would be really interested in finding out about your problems and how they are affecting your life. This might help us to think up some new ways to help, or we may just understand what is going on a bit better.*"

Notice how this emphasizes that the principal aim of the CBM is simply to understand problems better.

> "*Some people find helpful to look at their problems from a different perspective – perhaps we could see if it makes any sense to you.*"

This alleviates any pressure for the approach to 'succeed'. Trying out the CBM should be a 'no-lose' strategy, which avoids any sense of blame – for either GP or patient – if the approach proves unhelpful.

> "*This involves talking through all of the different aspects of your problems. You might also discover some new ways to cope better with your particular difficulties.*"

It is helpful to include a brief explanation of the CBM by describing how thoughts, feelings and behaviour are interrelated. You could discuss an example of how people may react differently to the same situation, such as the friend who was late for dinner in Chapter 2.

In the following dialogue, a GP gives a brief explanation and rationale for the CBM to a patient:

GP It is often helpful to look at your particular reactions to the difficulties in your life, since not everyone responds in the same way. Then it becomes possible to change any reactions that are unhelpful or making your problems worse. Let me give you an example: Imagine you have prepared dinner for a friend. An hour after she was due to arrive, there is no sign of her and you have had no phone call. How would you react to this?

Patient I would be really annoyed if she just didn't bother to turn up like that.

GP Absolutely. If you thought to yourself, 'How dare she do this to me – she is so rude not to bother to turn up!' you would almost certainly feel angry or annoyed. And you might react by telling her off once she did arrive or being cool with her.

Still, not everyone will have that exact same reaction. Someone else might see things very differently. Suppose another person thought to themselves, 'She didn't come because she doesn't really like me. She probably thinks I am too boring.' How might that person feel?

Patient Well, I suppose they would feel quite fed up and low.

GP Exactly right. Thinking like that would probably make you feel rather depressed and sad. Now, how do you think that person would behave if they thought that?

Patient I'm not sure.

GP Well, If someone thinks to themselves, 'I am really boring and no one likes me,' do you think they are likely to keep on inviting people over to dinner?

Patient No, they probably wouldn't bother to invite people at all.

GP That's right. They would stop inviting people over and they might stop going out so often. And when people become more isolated and alone, how do you think they would feel then?

Patient They would probably feel even more depressed and lonely.

GP Yes, by becoming isolated, that person starts to feel even worse in a kind of vicious cycle.

Patient I see – that makes sense.

GP Another person might think, 'Oh no... she's probably been in an accident. The roads are very dangerous these days' and feel very anxious, and yet another might think, 'Oh well, she's probably stuck in traffic' and feel calm and react by continuing to prepare dinner.

Now, can you see any way that this way of looking at things might apply to you and your problems?

Patient Well, I know I do tend to see things very negatively. I would always think the worst in a situation like that.

GP For some people, it is helpful to try to work out the kinds of thoughts, feelings and behaviours that make up their reactions to various situations. Would you be interested in looking at one or two of your problems in that way?

Patient Yes, I think that would be really interesting.

Notice how the GP actively involves the patient in the dialogue, rather than simply giving a monologue of information. This acts as an introduction to the CBM and begins to assess whether a particular patient would be interested in finding more about the approach.

Background reading for patients

It is often helpful to give patients some background reading. This educates and involves the patient in the CBM process, which is likely to make it more effective. By asking the patient to read the information and return, it also

From Theory to Practice...	Think up an example of different reactions to the same situation, similar to the dialogue above.
	Try using this example to explain the CBM to one or two patients. Remember to use open questions to keep the patient involved in the discussion.
	You may also choose to give the patient some CBT-related background reading.
	Ask the patient to return on another occasion to tell you their views on the approach.

identifies whether the patient is motivated to become actively involved in the process. This is a key indicator that it is more likely to be useful.

It is often helpful to give patients a relevant introductory leaflet about CBT (see Chapter 16 for suggestions of useful material):

> "*Would you be prepared have a look at this leaflet and then come back and tell me whether you think this approach might be helpful for you, and how?*"

Working Through the Stages of the CBM

The CBM is composed of five interrelated areas: thoughts, feelings, physical reactions/symptoms, behaviour and environmental factors.

Ideally, the information gathered through the CBM should be in a *written* format (see *Figure 4.1*)

Figure 4.1: CBM chart to use in consultations

Thoughts	Feelings
Behaviour	**Physical symptoms/biology**
Environmental factors/triggers	

Patients often reply to questions with a mixture of information from different areas of the CBM. For example, when asked for feelings, they may reply with thoughts. Rather than correcting the patient, it is more helpful to simply listen to the patient carefully and annotate the CBM chart with the relevant information in the appropriate section. When summarizing the information back to the patient, try to then break it down into the five areas.

Beginning the discussion

It is usually helpful to begin by talking about the area that the patient is already focussed on as their presenting complaint. For example, if a patient is complaining of feeling very anxious and panicky then the GP might say:

> "*You've mentioned that you feel very anxious and panicky sometimes. I am going to write that down on this chart. OK, now I would like to talk about some of the*

ways that you think and react when you feel so anxious. Can you give me a recent example of when you felt like this...?"

Focusing initially on the most important or worrying aspect of problems shows the patient that you are interested in what they see as the major problem and helps to build trust. This will facilitate the later exploration of other aspects of the problem such as emotional or cognitive factors, which the patient may not initially view as being relevant. This is particularly important in problems like health anxiety, where the patient is very fixed on one particular aspect of their problem – their physical symptoms. In this case, it is helpful to begin by reviewing the physical symptoms which are causing concern.

Reminders: Starting to work through the five areas of the CBM

- Give patients a clear explanation and rationale for using the CBM
- Use an example, such as a friend being late for dinner, to illustrate relationships between thoughts, feelings and behaviours
- Background reading gives will help the patient make better use of the CBM and helps identify whether the patient is motivated to use the model
- Begin by discussing the area of the CBM that the patient initially presents with
- Use a written CBM chart to record thoughts, feelings and behaviours

Eliciting thoughts

Thoughts play a key role in understanding problems using the CBM (*Figure 4.2*). Accurately understanding a person's thoughts is central to understanding their reactions to particular situations and events. This identifies the *meaning* of the event for that individual.

Figure 4.2: Role of thoughts in the CBM

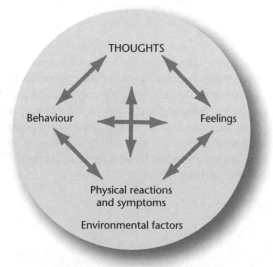

Be specific in recording thoughts and worries, by asking for recent examples of problems, e.g. a recent panic attack or a time when the patient felt really low.

"*What was going through your mind when you felt so anxious?*"

"*What is the worst bit about this? What is it about the situation that really gets to you?*"

Thoughts should reflect the patient's key emotions (and vice versa) and this relationship should make logical sense to the listener. If you don't quite feel you fully understand, continue to gently ask questions:

"*I would like to understand but I'm not quite with you. Can you explain...?*"

It is particularly important to use an appropriate questioning style, which avoids turning into an aggressive interrogation. Notice how the above statement and question avoids this by openly admitting to a lack of understanding and making a request to the patient to help enlighten the GP. Adopting an attitude of genuine interest in discovering more about problems will often generate a similar enthusiasm in the patient, which encourages them to address important problems.

Box 4.1:
Questions to help identify negative automatic thoughts

- What was going through your mind...? What were you thinking?
- What is the worst bit about this situation? What is so bad about it?
- What does this say about yourself, your life or your future?
- How do you see yourself, your behaviour or your performance?
- Were you afraid that something might happen? What would be the worst thing?
- How do you think others thought or felt about you in that situation? What does that mean to you?
- Did you have any particular memories or images?

It is important to use the patient's *own words* when recording thoughts. This makes the discussion feel more relevant and real for the patient. Particular words or phrases often have very specific and powerful meanings to individuals. By changing what they say to a more 'medicalized' version, the discussion may not resonate with their actual experiences and you may lose the emotional connection with the patient. Remember also to use the *first person,* for example by writing "I am a failure" rather than "Thinking about being a failure."

Case example 4.1: Identifying thoughts

Alison is a 25-year old hairdresser who has been suffering from stress and anxiety for six months. She used to be part of a big group of friends, but has recently become anxious about spending time with them. She has begun avoiding meeting large groups of people, and has therefore become more isolated in her daily life.

GP You said that you felt very anxious just before you were due to go and meet your friends. Can you tell me what was going through your mind at that moment?

Alison I was thinking that I didn't want to go because the whole evening would probably be a disaster.

GP What were you concerned might happen to make the whole evening a disaster?

Alison Well, I might say something really stupid in front of the group, or I might not say anything at all.

GP Supposing that did happen – that you said something stupid in front of the group, or you didn't have anything to say – what would be so bad about that? What would it mean about you or what others think of you?

Alison I suppose it might mean that my friends would laugh at me. They might think less of me. And if I don't say anything at all, they would think I am boring.

GP OK, I would like to summarize what I heard you say. The situation was that last Thursday evening you were due to meet some friends. Before going out, you were feeling very anxious and you were thinking: 'I don't want to go. The whole evening might be a disaster. I might say something stupid in front of the group or not say anything at all. My friends might laugh at me and think less of me. If I don't say anything they will think I am boring.' Is that right? Is there anything you would like to add or change?

Alison That's right. I hadn't really thought of it like that before. It made me feel really tense and uptight before I went out.

GP Could you tell me which one of these thoughts is the most powerful or upsetting? Which is the 'hot' thought?

Alison Well… I think the most upsetting thought is that '*My friends might laugh at me and think less of me.*'

GP OK, that's very useful to know. We will draw a circle around that thought.

Notice how the GP simply listened and recorded Alison's thoughts, word for word, *without* trying to question or challenge them. Once both Alison and the GP fully understand all five areas of the CBM in relation to this problem, only then is it helpful to start to look at challenging or re-framing thoughts.

Reminders: Eliciting thoughts

■ Identifying automatic thoughts, memories and images helps understand the meaning of an event for an individual person
■ Be genuinely interested in understanding deeply but avoid interrogating the patient
■ Use the patient's own words when recording and discussing their thoughts
■ Identify the 'hot thought' which is associated with the strongest feelings and emotions

From Theory to Practice...	Make a note of some key questions to ask patients about their thoughts. Then try them out with one or two patients. You may sometimes be surprised at the answers you receive!
	These questions are a good way to understand more about patients' experiences even without discussing all five areas of the CBM.

Discussing feelings

It is important to identify the feelings that cause a patient's major emotional distress. Try to stay focused and relate feelings to specific thoughts and situations:

"When you start to think ... how does that make you feel?"

"How did you feel in that situation...?"

If you simply wish to gain a broad understanding of the patient's feelings and other experiences, it is sometimes helpful to take a more general approach:

"Can you tell me a bit about how you are generally and how you are feeling?"

Patients are not always able to easily articulate their feelings. Some may find it difficult to admit or express feelings, or may simply be less aware of them than others. If patients have difficulty identifying their feelings, one option is to suggest a likely *opposite* reaction:

"Did you feel very happy and relaxed in that situation?"

The patient is likely to respond quickly to correct the 'error': e.g. "Oh no, I felt really stressed and uptight."

This opens up the discussion and gives the GP an opportunity to discuss the thoughts and behaviours associated with the particular feeling.

"What was going through your mind that was making you feel stressed and uptight?"

As a last resort, if a patient is really struggling to identify their feelings, the clinician can make one or two suggestions. However, you must also accept that these are *guesses* and may be inaccurate for a particular individual.

"Some people find that this kind of situation makes them feel fed up or down, could that be true for you? If not, what might be more accurate?"

"I could imagine that thinking 'I am such a failure' might make someone feel very low. Is that true for you?"

You can also reflect back to patients any particular feelings that you have observed. Again, it is important to be flexible and be aware that you may have incorrectly labelled a particular feeling.

"This pain really seems to make you angry."

"You seem very sad and low when you say that."

It is always important to express empathy for the patient's unpleasant feelings and experiences:

"It sounds really difficult to feel that way. It must be very unpleasant to feel so anxious."

Reminders: Identifying feelings

- Identify the feelings associated with specific situations and thoughts
- Suggesting the *opposite* reaction can be helpful if patients have difficulty identifying feelings
- Express empathy for unpleasant, negative feelings and emotions

Looking at behaviour

It is important to spend time identifying a patient's helpful and unhelpful behaviours and coping strategies and how these relate to other areas of the CBM (*Figure 4.3*).

Figure 4.3: Role of behaviour in CBM

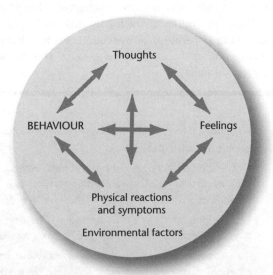

Begin by simply asking the patient how they behave in particular situations:

"What happens when you feel anxious? What do you do then?"

It is often helpful to ask the patient to compare their current behaviour to that of other times in their lives or to other people's reactions:

"What are you doing differently now that you feel so low? How was life before this? What did you do then?"

"How might you behave differently if you felt happier and more relaxed?"

"Do you know anyone else who would react differently in this situation? What would they do?"

It is sometimes useful to discuss the specific thoughts and fears that underlie certain behaviours. This helps to make sense of reactions which may initially seem self-defeating and difficult to understand.

"What is the worst thing that could happen if you hadn't taken that action to cope with your symptoms?"

"What makes you react that way? What might happen if you didn't?"

The patient must be encouraged to generate their *own* solutions and strategies for changing unhelpful behaviour. This helps to avoid the classic, 'Yes, but...' responses to suggestions made by GPs.

If patients do try out new behaviour, it is also useful for them to make a note of what happened, ideally in a written journal. For example, did they feel better or worse than before? This highlights any improvement, no matter how small, and serves as a useful reminder on days that people are feeling discouraged or low.

Reminders: Looking at behaviour

■ Identify the patient's behaviour patterns, associated with different problems and situations
■ Ask about the thoughts and fears which may drive unhelpful behaviours
■ Encourage patients to generate their own strategies for changing behaviour
■ Monitoring and recording the effect of behavioural changes encourages patients to keep trying to change old habits

From Theory to Practice...	Remember to include questions about behaviour when discussing problems with patients.
	Try to discover *unhelpful* behaviours, which may worsen problems, as well as *helpful* coping strategies, which can be encouraged. What underlying thoughts, fears or beliefs are driving these behaviours?
	Try to look at the role of behaviour in one or two patients with psychological or emotional problems (e.g. depression or anxiety).
	Can you identify any unhelpful behaviour in one or two patients with physical disorders such as back pain or diabetes?

Reviewing physical symptoms

Concerns about physical symptoms often prompt people to attend GPs and it is important to spend time reviewing the patient's physical symptoms and reactions. Physical reactions can also play an important role in the CBM, particularly where unhelpful beliefs exist about the *meaning* of symptoms, such as in panic attacks or health anxiety.

> "*I would like to briefly review how this is affecting you physically. Can you remind me which physical symptoms you commonly experience?*"

It can be useful to identify the physical reactions of the patient during a particular situation or associated with a particular feeling.

> "*How did you feel physically at that time when you were so anxious? What bodily sensations were you aware of?*"

In health anxiety, it is important to listen empathically and simply record what the patient says *without* trying to explain symptoms or minimize how important or distressing they may be. This may generate a relatively long list of symptoms. However, getting into debates about the significance, severity or meaning of a particular symptom will simply lengthen the discussion and detract focus from the main aim of the discussion: to understand and record the physical experiences of that patient.

> "*OK, so you have headaches and neck pain. Are there any other symptoms?*"
>
> "*It helps me to get an overview of all of your different symptoms.*"

Remember to listen and express empathy for any unpleasant or distressing physical experiences.

> "*It must be really distressing to feel so much pain.*"

Once you have generated a list of physical symptoms, finish by asking the patient to identify the one or two most distressing symptoms and put a circle around them.

> "*Which symptom is the most severe or bothers you the most?*"

The next stage is to identify the patient's underlying fears and beliefs about the meaning of their symptoms.

> "*Can you give me a recent example of when the pain in your back was really severe and bothered you? What was the most distressing part about experiencing the pain?*"
>
> "*What do you think that having this headache means? Do you have any thoughts about what might be causing it?*"
>
> "*What went through your mind when you noticed the tightness in your chest?*"

It is important to understand the unique impact of particular symptoms on a patient's life. This includes fears about *future* changes.

> "*How do these symptoms affect your life? What do these changes mean to you or about you? How does that make you feel emotionally?*"

"Are you concerned that something may change or worsen in the future?"

Negative thoughts or beliefs about how to respond to particular symptoms may also result in unhelpful behaviours, such as excessive resting with back pain.

"How do you react when you experience this symptom? What might happen if you did not?"

Try to finish with a summary of the physical symptoms and any related thoughts and feelings. This highlights the links between physical and psychological aspects of problems *without* suggesting that physical symptoms are 'all in the patient's mind' and not 'real'.

"You mentioned that you are experiencing some very unpleasant symptoms, which are making your life really difficult. You are suffering from headaches, dizziness and occasional tingling in the feet. The dizziness is the most unpleasant symptom. You had a bout of dizziness yesterday, and when it happened, you began to think: 'Maybe I have got a brain tumour,' which made you feel very anxious."

Reminders: Reviewing physical symptoms

■ Generate a comprehensive list of the patient's physical symptoms
■ Ask the patient to identify one or two most important or severe symptoms
■ Spend time identifying patients' underlying beliefs and fears about the *meaning* of physical symptoms, as well as associated behavioural reactions
■ End by with a brief summary, which highlights any links between key physical symptoms, thoughts, feelings and behaviours

From Theory to Practice...	Choose one or two patients with distressing physical symptoms: • Review their symptoms and identify any underlying fears and beliefs about the meaning of symptoms. How does experiencing the symptoms affect the patient's life? Do they fear that this could change or worsen in the future? • What kinds of feelings are associated with these thoughts? Does this affect how the patient behaves?

Including social and environmental factors

It is important to identify relevant social and environmental stressors, which may contribute to the patient's difficulties. It is useful to give patients a rationale for asking about personal life circumstances:

"It may help to understand anything going on in your life which may be making you feel upset and making your symptoms worse."

Make sure you discuss all possible relevant social, environmental and cultural factors (*Box 4.2*).

Box 4.2:

Important social and environmental factors

- Are there problems with any important relationships (family, friends, neighbours)?
- Do you have enough support?
- Do you have someone to talk to about problems?
- Are there demands at home, such as looking after children or other relatives?
- Are there money troubles?
- Are there any particular problems with housing or the home environment?
- Are you unemployed or unable to work?
- Are there difficulties at work?

It may also be important to identify and understand whether particular situations act as triggers for problems:

> "*Do the panic attacks arise in any specific situations?*"

> "*What is it about this situation that you find so difficult? What is the worst thing that could happen?*"

Some environments are so challenging, it would be difficult for anyone to maintain a positive outlook. For example, a person being abused by a family member is likely to need help to either change or leave the situation. However, sometimes patients may feel unable or choose not to change difficult situations such as these. This can be frustrating and distressing for health professionals, who wish the best for their patients.

In these cases, it is useful to focus on helping the patient to cope with the difficult circumstances, rather than judging the patient or labelling them as 'impossible to help'. Working on negative self-beliefs, such as improving a patient's low self-esteem, could also be a relevant precursor to making difficult life changes.

Problem-solving techniques can be used to make changes in environmental problems (see Chapter 9).

Reminders: Social and environmental factors

- Identify key environmental and social factors that are having a negative impact on the patient's health and well-being
- Look for environmental triggers for disorders such as panic attacks
- Problem-solving strategies are useful for changing practical problems
- It may sometimes be useful to focus on helping patients to cope with adverse situations

Chapter 5

Consultation skills for the CBM

- Identifying and learning specific consultation *skills* teaches GPs *how* to implement the CBM in practice

- The skills encourage a structured and focused approach to consultations, which makes the most effective use of limited time

- By using these consultation skills, GPs can empower patients to take responsibility for finding new solutions and coping strategies for their problems

Why focus on consultation skills?

Identifying and learning the specific consultation skills needed for the CBM (*Box 5.1*) teaches us *how* to apply the model in practice. The skills help to use the CBM effectively within the brief time available in most GP consultations. The vast majority of GPs are *already* highly practised communicators and the skills for the CBM simply build on any GP's existing skills and knowledge.

Box 5.1: Key consultation skills for use with the CBM

1. Writing down relevant information
2. Agenda setting
3. Focus on specific and concrete issues
4. Cognitive empathy
5. Collaboration (working in partnership)
6. Obtaining feedback
7. Link-making
8. Setting and reviewing homework

Writing down relevant information

Using the CBM is most effective if all information gathered is written down, with one copy kept for the GP's records and another given to the patient. There should be open discussion about whatever the GP writes down. Patients may feel uncomfortable or suspicious if they are unable to see what is being written. It is therefore ideal to sit with a piece of paper positioned between clinician and patient, with both able to see it clearly. This enables the GP to summarize the patient's words easily, whilst pointing at the relevant parts of the model.

There are several reasons for writing relevant information down:

- It helps patients to remember key points from the consultation.

- Seeing their own words in 'black-and-white' helps patients to disassociate from their problems and gain a broader perspective. This encourages more flexible thinking about difficulties, as if they belonged to someone else.

- A written overview highlights any links between different areas of patients' problems. It is useful to physically draw the links between areas of the CBM as arrows on the paper.

- Writing down information slows down the process of information gathering and gives the consultation more structure and focus.

- The GP is able to relax and focus on listening.

- Written notes also enable the GP to reflect back accurate summaries of the information, using the patient's own words.

Begin by explaining that you plan to write down the key points and the reasons for this:

> *"It is very important to me to accurately remember what you say, so I would like write down the main points. We can discuss whatever I write and you can take away a copy of the information after the consultation. Are you happy for me to take some notes?"*

It is often helpful to use writing information down as an opportunity to summarize and check back with the patient that you understand them correctly.

> *"You said that you felt 'hurt' and 'angry' – I am going to write that down. Is that OK?"*

You can also use this to clarify important points:

> *"Right – you have given me lots of information here which seems important to note down. Before moving on, let's just check back over the key points..."*

Some GPs may feel uncomfortable about using written records in this way. Computer systems may not enable the input of such detailed information. To overcome this, some GPs keep a folder of CBM charts/patient information which they hold separately or scan into the patient's computerized notes. They minimize duplication by making a brief computer entry, such as 'Discussion about feelings of depression using CBT' and any particular outcomes or treatment issued.

Some beliefs held by GPs may hinder the use of written information, such as:

> *"If I spend too much time writing, the patient will think it is rude."*
>
> *"Writing will interfere with good communication with the patient."*
>
> *"I don't have time to write things down."*
>
> *"I can remember what the patient says – I don't need to write anything down."*

Many of these beliefs can be challenged and reframed. For example, the patient may *not* think the GP is rude to look away on occasions in order to write what they say down, provided the GP offers an explanation for what they are doing, involves the patient in what is being written and maintains good eye-contact in between making notes.

Writing can facilitate *better* communication with patients, provided it is used in a sensitive, open and collaborative way. Unless you have an unbelievably good memory, it is rarely possible to accurately remember the precise information given by patients about complex problems.

Writing information may also help, rather than hinder, effective time management. The process of writing helps maintain focus on the important issues. Giving the patient a written record to consider after their brief GP appointment utilizes time outside the consultation as well.

Reminders: Writing information down

■ It is helpful to have a written record of any discussion using the CBM and to give a copy to patients afterwards
■ Visual records of information including links between different areas of problems can be very powerful
■ Writing information helps add structure and maintain focus of consultations
■ Writing aids recall and encourages use of the patient's own words when summarizing information

From Theory to Practice...	Have a go at writing a patient's information down. Treat it as a 'behavioural experiment'.
	If you have any negative predictions or concerns about using written records, treat these thoughts as 'hypotheses' to be tested out in practice.
	Then, simply try it out on a few patients and take note of the outcome.

Agenda setting

Setting an agenda involves spending a short period at the beginning of the consultation negotiating how the time should be used. The aim is to:

• Ensure that the patient's key issues are covered during the consultation or deferred for a later stage

• Optimize the use of limited time by devoting greater time to the most important issues

• Improve GP–patient partnership by encouraging the patient to take the lead in setting the agenda.

Setting an agenda can help the patient to prioritize the most important issues to cover in a consultation. Patients often have as many as five or more items that they would like to discuss per consultation (Barry *et al.*, 2000). However, it may be impossible to cover all these items during only ten minutes. An open discussion about time constraints can reduce the pressure to cover more than is realistically possible in one appointment.

"As we have limited time, I would like to spend a moment checking what you would like to discuss today, to make sure we cover what is most important to you."

"We may not have time to cover everything but we can come back to anything important that we miss at another time."

As part of a collaborative doctor–patient partnership, the GP can also place items on the agenda.

"I would also like us to look at some new ways for you to deal with your anxiety symptoms. Would that be of interest to you?"

It is helpful to use the agenda to maintain focus if discussions have drifted away from agreed areas. Responsibility for sticking to the agenda can be shared between patient and doctor.

"We agreed earlier that we would spend today talking about… I've noticed that we have moved away from that and I'm concerned there will not be enough time to cover the areas you felt were most important. What should we do – continue as we are or get back to the agenda?"

Having an agenda can also help to close the discussion towards the end of the consultation.

"As we discussed at the beginning of the consultation, we do have limited time today and unfortunately we are nearing the end of the appointment. Perhaps we could finish by checking whether we covered what was on the agenda…"

Case example 5.1: Setting an agenda

John is a 45-year old IT manager who has presented to his GP on several occasions with increasing anxiety and low mood.

GP Hello John, how are things?

John Not very good, I'm afraid. I'm still feeling terrible. We are having all kinds of problems with our son, Andrew. Work is pretty stressful too. There seem to be so many problems right now; I don't know how to deal with them all.

GP Oh dear, I'm sorry to hear that things are so tough for you. It sounds really difficult. Perhaps we could spend some time talking through some of these issues. As our time is limited, what is the most important problem to talk about today?

John I'm not sure. There are so many difficult things…

GP That's true. But we could make a note of what we don't cover and come back to it next time. You mentioned that you are feeling terrible and also that you are concerned about your son and that work is stressful. Should we look at one of these areas today or is there something else…?

John I think the worst thing is that I am feeling so anxious and low at the moment. It affects every other part of my life.

GP Ok, that sounds like a good place to start.

John Yes, I think so.

Reminders: Agenda setting

■ Setting an agenda optimizes the use of limited time by identifying the most important issues to discuss

■ GP and patient work in partnership to set and stick to agendas

■ An agenda can help maintain a relevant, focused discussion during the consultation

From Theory to Practice...	Try collaboratively setting a brief agenda in one or two consultations, particularly with patients who usually present with multiple or complex issues.
	Make sure you do not spend too much of the consultation time setting the agenda itself!
	What is the impact of setting an agenda on (a) the doctor and (b) the patient?

Focus on specific and concrete areas

Using a focused approach to problems is a key feature of the CBM. Patients do sometimes benefit from the opportunity to simply 'offload' and talk about their problems in a safe environment. However, an unstructured discussion can sometimes result in both patient and doctor feeling overwhelmed and confused.

The CBM encourages patients to break down their problems into manageable 'chunks'. One of the first steps is to focus on one important area at a time. This process begins by negotiating an agenda. The next step is to look at specific areas of the problem. Maintaining focus helps the patient to concentrate on the most important issues.

The CBM uses an open, focussed approach by using open questions to explore key issues in depth. Staying focussed can be seen as *vertical* as opposed to *horizontal* discussion about problems – it enables the patient to dig below the surface and explore their problems more deeply.

One of the most effective ways to keep focused is to ask the patient for recent, concrete examples of specific incidents:

> *"Could you give me a recent example of a situation where you felt very anxious? What happened?"*

The first step is to identify the details of the situation: when, where, who, what? It is helpful to discover at what exact point during the situation the patient began to feel anxious. This technique is like using a microscope to examine a very brief moment in time – the point at which a negative feeling suddenly became very strong. During this short period, it is likely that the key negative automatic thoughts to explain the reaction can be identified.

> *"At exactly what point did you start to feel bad?"*
>
> *"What were you doing?"*
>
> *"At that moment, what was running through your mind?"*

The tone of voice and style of questioning is critically important to gain patients' trust. For example, asking repeated *'Why...?'* questions can appear aggressive or threatening. Feeling defensive will also make people less open to learning new ways to think about situations. More helpful questions include:

"How...?"

"Tell me about...?"

"I'm not quite with you. Could you explain...?"

It is important to convey a genuine interest in exploring any patient's problems. Try to see the process as a 'voyage of discovery' into a patient's psychological and emotional life. After all, the information generated is often genuinely fascinating. This attitude also encourages patients to become interested in understanding and solving their problems.

Case example 5.2: Taking a focused approach to problems

The following dialogue continues the discussion between John, a 45-year old IT manager, and his GP, which began above.

GP   OK, when we were setting the agenda, you said that it was most important to discuss the way you are feeling so anxious and low at the moment.

John   Yes, that's right. I am feeling so anxious and down. I never used to be like this.

GP   I see. That must be very distressing for you. I would like to understand more about how this is affecting you. Can you think of an example of a situation in the past week or so when you felt like this?

John   Yes, there were many occasions.

GP   It can often be useful to focus on one specific time that you felt bad. Can you think a recent, 'typical' example?

John   Err... Yesterday when I was given a deadline at work to finish a report.

GP   [*Writing the information*]   Yesterday, when you were given a deadline?

John   Yes

GP   Can you tell me at what exact point you started to feel anxious and low? What were you doing then?

John   I started to feel anxious as soon as I sat down at my computer to start the report.

GP   OK, that's very helpful. Is that a typical situation that you might feel anxious?

John   Yes, I find it really difficult at work at the moment.

GP   Let's talk about it in a bit more depth...

Reminders: Focus on specific and concrete areas

- Use open questions about specific areas to generate information about key issues
- Ask for specific, recent examples of incidents which illustrate the patient's problem(s)
- Remember to convey a genuine interest in exploring the patient's problems

From Theory to Practice...	Try asking one or two patients for a specific and concrete example of when they experienced a particular problem.
	Notice the level and depth of information they can generate about specific incidents.
	How relevant or useful is the information gathered? Can it be generalized to understand the patient as a whole? How does this process affect the flow, amount or type of information generated in the consultation?

Cognitive empathy

Cognitive empathy involves understanding what *really matters* to a patient, without assuming, guessing or generalizing. There are many different ways of reacting to the same situation. Health professionals should never assume they understand why a patient may experience emotional distress in any particular set of circumstances.

Offering genuine empathy for the specific thoughts, feelings and behaviours that contribute towards a distressing situation is far more powerful than general platitudes or expressions of sympathy. The clinician must attempt to understand the patient's inner experience, by trying to "step into the patient's world and see and experience life the way the patient does" (Beck *et al.*, 1979: 24). This is more than simply reassuring patients that they are being heard and understood, and implies understanding the cognitive basis for the feelings as well as the emotions themselves.

A cognitively empathic GP understands how the patient's thinking leads to specific feelings and behaviours, but *does not need to agree with the thinking* if it is illogical or exacerbates rather than resolves problems. Nevertheless it is essential to accept that the patient's thoughts and feelings seem valid to them and should not be dismissed or belittled.

Expressing cognitive empathy involves making appropriate empathic statements based on the information you have gathered:

> "*It must feel really scary if you think 'It must be cancer' every time you get the pain.*"

> "*You sounded really upset just then.*"

Cognitive empathy is about being interested in the patient's view of the world. It can be very rewarding for the GP, who is in the privileged position of being able to share a great deal of personal information from people's lives. Many GPs find this one of the most fascinating parts of general practice.

Case example 5.3: Cognitive empathy

Maureen is a 40-year old woman who has been depressed for about six months. Her mother died of a heart attack three years earlier whilst on the telephone to Maureen. She has recently become preoccupied by guilt that she was unable to do anything to prevent the death of her mother.

Compare the following two scenarios. Look carefully at the questions used by the doctor and the responses of the patient:

- What kinds of questions and statements are used by the GP? How do these affect Maureen's responses?
- Does the GP show *sympathy* or *cognitive empathy*? What impact does this have?
- How do you think Maureen felt during and after this consultation?
- Which consultation do you think the GP would find most interesting and rewarding?

Scenario A:

Maureen My mother had a heart attack while on the phone to me. I feel so bad, I should have been able to do something.
GP What a terrible thing to happen! That sounds really traumatic.
Maureen Yes it was really awful.
GP And how are you feeling now?
Maureen I really feel terrible, so guilty.
GP Yes, you poor thing. It's quite understandable to feel that way. I think many people would feel like that under the circumstances.
Maureen I'm really sure it's all my fault.
GP I don't think it really is your fault. But it is common and quite normal to feel that way after a big shock. It's all part of the grief reaction.
Maureen I just don't know what to do. I feel so terrible.
GP Most people find that things do get better with time.

In this example, the GP was caring and sympathetic towards Maureen's difficulties but failed to explore *why* Maureen felt so upset. After some good initial empathic statements and an open question (*"How are you feeling now?"*), the GP then resorted to a prescriptive statement (*"It is normal to feel that way."*). Whilst it can sometimes be helpful to 'normalize' a patient's feelings, at this point in the discussion, the GP cannot really be sure whether Maureen is suffering from a 'normal' grief reaction or whether her feelings relate to another problem, such as worsening depression. Maureen may have appreciated the GP's sympathy but it seems unlikely that she would feel better about the problem after this consultation.

Scenario B:

Maureen My mother had a heart attack while on the phone to me. I feel so bad, I should have been able to do something

continued

GP That sounds like a really awful experience. Tell me what happened...

Maureen Well, we were chatting and she suddenly said, "Maureen, I feel strange" and then gasped and went silent. I phoned my brother who lives nearby. He went round straight away but she was already dead.

GP You said that you feel really bad about it?

Maureen Yes, it's all my fault.

GP Tell me how you came to that conclusion?

Maureen Earlier in the week, mum had said that she wasn't feeling well. I offered to take her to the doctor but she said she thought it was a cold and would settle on its own. If only I'd insisted on taking her – she might never have had the heart attack.

GP So you feel bad because you didn't insist on taking her to the doctor earlier in the week?

Maureen Yes, I let her down.

GP I see. It must be really difficult to feel so bad and to believe that you let your mother down.

Maureen It is difficult. If only I had realized she was seriously ill.

GP Tell me Maureen, did you know it was her heart, when you were talking to your mother earlier in the week?

Maureen No, I thought it was just a cold, like she said. She often got them.

GP If you had known it was her heart, would you have behaved differently?

Maureen Oh yes, I would definitely have taken her to the doctor if I had known that.

GP But you didn't know?

Maureen No, I didn't.

GP Hmmm, I wonder what advice you might give to a friend in the same situation?

Maureen I suppose I would say that she's blaming herself for something she just didn't know would happen.

GP How do you tie that together with your idea that you let your mother down for not preventing her heart attack?

Maureen I suppose I really couldn't have known what would happen, it's not like I deliberately ignored something serious.

In this example, the GP takes time to explore exactly what was making Maureen feel so guilty and upset about the death of her mother. The GP demonstrates cognitive empathy in several key questions. When Maureen says she is convinced that the death of her mother is her fault, the GP asks: *"Tell me how you came to that conclusion?"* This opens the discussion to explore Maureen's view of the problem. The GP also makes several empathic statements based on Maureen's description of her thoughts and feelings.

After understanding Maureen's key thoughts and feelings, the GP gently encourages her to look at the situation from a new perspective. The GP does not tell Maureen what to think, but uses Maureen's own knowledge and experience to encourage her to find her own answers. Whilst it may not have solved Maureen's problems, the discussion may have given her some new perspectives and strengthened the relationship with her GP.

Reminders: Cognitive empathy

■ Cognitive empathy involves trying to understand the patient's view of their world
■ Make empathic statements based on the specific thoughts, feelings and behaviours that contribute towards patients' distress

From Theory to Practice...	Try not to jump to conclusions about why people may be upset or suffering from emotional distress. Take time to fully explore their view of the situation – it can be a fascinating process!

Developing collaboration and partnership

Collaboration involves building a partnership where the GP and patient *work together as a team* to understand problems, set goals and develop solutions. A collaborative relationship enables the patient to discover new perspectives for problems themselves, rather than being convinced or persuaded by the GP.

GPs can work with the patient against a third 'party' – the patient's *problem(s)* – rather than focusing on changing the *patient*. This emphasis on solving problems rather than on a patient's 'faults' or 'defects' reduces any sense of shame, inadequacy or defensiveness, and helps patients to work more effectively to bring about changes.

The communication style of the GP has an important role in developing collaborative relationships with patients. The GP needs to use a flexible, negotiating style, and avoid playing 'absolute expert'. This involves being open to the patient's suggestions, following their lead, and being prepared to acknowledge and deal with any misunderstandings or mistakes. It is also important to explain all procedures and treatment approaches openly and jointly carry out processes such as setting an agenda and agreeing homework.

Using guided discovery to build collaboration

The process of guided discovery enables GP and patient to explore problems together. It is like a 'dance' where the GP follows the lead of the patient in discovering what is important or relevant to each individual as an expert in their own lives.

The GP's role is to support the patient and help them to focus on the most important issues. This involves clarifying, summarizing and reflecting back key information to the patient. The shared approach of guided discovery is empowering for the patient and reduces pressure on the GP to provide answers that they may not actually possess.

Reminders: Collaboration and guided discovery

- GP and patient should work together as a *team* to understand and solve problems
- Keep a flexible style, follow the patient's lead and avoid playing 'absolute expert'
- Guided discovery is a way to jointly explore problems that encourages the patient to take responsibility for finding their own solutions

The stages of guided discovery (Padesky, 2003)

1. Asking informational questions

Begin by asking informational questions to discover more about each area of the CBM. These questions should begin with general, open questions to establish the patient's main areas of concern:

"Tell me about ... "

"How does that affect you...?"

To clarify important information, use more focused and specific questions.

"Can you give me an example?"

"What was it about that situation which really bothered you...?"

"What does being unable to work mean for you?"

Don't be afraid to keep gently 'digging' to clarify exactly what the patient means.

2. Empathic listening

Good listening is central to all effective communication. In primary care consultations, patients often express important information as 'cues', which may be missed if the health professional is not listening carefully. Empathic listening is important in the 'dance' of guided discovery. It enables the GP to follow the lead of the patient. As emphasized above, making written notes can also promote effective listening.

3. Summarizing

Summarizing is one of the most important skills for the CBM. Summaries form a natural break in consultations which give the patient an opportunity to reflect upon what they have said. Patients need time and space in order to make cognitive and emotional changes.

Make frequent summaries, ideally every few sentences and written down. Wherever possible, use the patient's own words.

"When your boss asked to see you, you thought 'I'm going to lose my job. How will I be able to pay the mortgage? We could lose our home,' and you felt very anxious and worried."

Summaries encourage patients to view their problems from a new perspective, which may be more objective. They also show the patient that they have been listened to and that their perspective is understood. This helps to build a good relationship between GP and patient and also helps to prevent or correct any misunderstandings.

Brief summaries should be used frequently as reflective statements:

"So when you get the pain, you think 'I'll never get better,' and that makes you feel down and low?"

It is also useful to include one or two detailed summaries, which bring together information gathered over a period of time:

"I'd like to summarize what we talked about today. You told me that the panic attacks are getting worse and are starting to affect your work – you now avoid some situations, such as giving presentations. You gave me an example of a panic attack last week, when you were about to speak to a group of colleagues. You started feeling anxious and you were thinking: 'What if I have another panic attack? I might make a complete fool of myself.' Physically you noticed that your heart was racing, your hands were sweaty and your chest felt tight. And then you thought to yourself, 'It's not normal to feel this bad. Maybe this means there is something wrong with my heart.' This made you feel even more panicky. You reacted by making an excuse to leave the room and cancelled the meeting. Does that seem accurate to you?"

4. Synthesizing questions

This is a crucial stage of guided discovery, which encourages the patient to take responsibility for making sense of their problems. It is often tempting for health professionals to offer solutions or explanations for a patient's problems, but this not the most effective way for patients to implement genuine changes in their life.

Instead, ask the patient to consider what they can learn or understand from the discussion:

"So…how do you tie all of this together?"

"What do you make of all this…?"

"Can you see any other way to view this situation…?"

"What might you say to a friend in the same situation…?"

A synthesizing question is a useful approach to take if the consultation has become 'stuck' and the GP feels uncertain how to proceed. Simply ask the patient what they make of the discussion so far. This can often be extremely interesting and enlightening. Being 'stuck' may also indicate that not enough time has been spent on fully understanding the key aspects of the problem.

Case example 5.4: Guided discovery

Let's return to John, the 45-year old IT manager suffering from anxiety and depression. In the previous dialogue, John identified a situation at work where he felt typically stressed and anxious.

In the following example, the GP explores John's problems with him. Read through the dialogue and try to identify each of the four stages of guided discovery:

continued

GP OK, imagine yourself back in that situation for a moment. You are sitting at your desk with a report to write that has a deadline. What was going through your mind at that moment?

John I was thinking 'I'll never get it done on time' and that 'It won't be good enough."

GP And if it wasn't good enough?

John If it wasn't good enough then I would look like a fool in front of my boss or might even lose my job.

GP I see. Can you tell me how you were feeling when you were thinking those things?

John Yes, I was feeling really anxious.

GP I see, feeling anxious. Were there any other strong feelings?

John Well, I was also feeling sad.

GP OK, can I check that I understand you? When you sat down at your computer to start the report, you started having some negative thoughts. You were thinking: 'I'll never get it done on time,' 'It won't be good enough' and 'I will look like a fool in front of my boss or might even lose my job.' And when you thought those things, you started feeling anxious and sad. Is that right, or is there something you would like me to correct?

John That's exactly how it was.

GP Oh dear. That sounds very unpleasant and stressful.

John Yes, it was really terrible.

GP Did you have any physical symptoms when you were feeling like that?

John Yes, I was feeling tense and sweaty. I started to get a headache.

GP I see. And how did you react in this situation? What did you do?

John I just sat there for a while. Then I couldn't face it anymore so I put off starting and started doing something else instead. Eventually I had to do the report but I left it so late that I had to rush through and I don't think it was very good.

GP OK, I've written down everything you told me. It seems like there may be a bit of a vicious cycle here. You said that you were thinking 'I'll never get it done' and 'it won't be good enough' and that made you feel anxious and sad. You reacted by putting off starting the report and then having to rush through it so it wasn't as good as you would have liked. Tell me, what do you make of all this we have been talking about?

John I can really see how I have got trapped in a cycle. The more worried and negative I feel about the report, the more I put off starting it, which makes me even more anxious and I have to rush the report.

GP Yes, that makes a lot of sense. Now that you have found this vicious cycle, maybe we could look at some ways to break it and maybe turn it into a more positive cycle. Do you have any thoughts how you might do this...?

Reminders: The four stages of guided discovery

1. *Asking informational questions*
   Open questions which focus on *specific* areas of the problem
2. *Empathic listening*
   Careful listening and expression of empathic statements based on the distressing thoughts and feelings described by patients
3. *Summarizing*
   Reflecting back information expressed by patients enables them to consider problems from a new perspective
4. *'Synthesizing' questions*
   Ties together relevant information and encourages the patient to make sense of problems themselves

From Theory to Practice...	Try to include some of the stages of guided discovery in your consultations. Don't try to do them all at once. Focus on each stage at a time.
	For example, try increasing the number of summaries you make in a consultation. On another occasion try asking a synthesizing question.
	What impact does this have on your consultation?

Obtaining feedback

Asking for regular feedback about the patient's view of the CBM process shows that their opinion is valued and important. This strengthens relationships with patients and increases their involvement in the consultation.

> "*It is very important for me to accurately understand your experiences. I would be like you to let me know if anything does not make sense or does not seem quite right to you. This will help us to work together on any problems.*"

Even when clinicians may wish to promote collaboration or partnership with patients, there may still be an imbalance of power where patients feel unable to question or challenge the authority of the doctor (Say & Thompson, 2003). Actively asking for feedback can help to overcome this barrier. It also enables the GP to check the patient's knowledge and attitude to the CBM process. This is also important since patients will not be used to GPs approaching problems in this way, and may be confused or have negative as well as positive reactions to the model.

> "*Could you tell me whether this approach makes sense to you? What do you make of it?*"

Asking for feedback naturally follows after the clinician gives a summary of the information so far.

> "*I'd like to check that I understand you correctly. You said that you often feel very depressed at the moment. One evening last week you started thinking 'I am a*

burden to my family' and decided not to make your usual visit to your mother. That evening you felt particularly down and lonely.

Is that right or am I not quite with you? Would something else be more accurate?"

The GP must be flexible enough to openly discuss and revise their view of any misunderstandings or mistakes highlighted by the patient. It is important to see obtaining feedback as a positive step that builds relationships and encourages mutual respect between clinician and patient.

Reminders: Obtaining feedback

- Asking for feedback gives the message that the patient's opinions are important and valued
- It is helpful to ask for feedback after giving a summary of the information so far
- The GP must be flexible enough to revise their opinion when necessary to correct any misunderstandings or mistakes that have arisen

Link-making

Identifying links between the five areas of the CBM helps to deepen a patient's understanding of how different aspects of individual problems are connected, and may help to identify potential solutions or areas for change. It is particularly helpful to identify any *vicious cycles* that are maintaining or worsening problems.

Making links can be a subtle process, which simply reflects and summarizes information presented by patients:

"You mentioned that you were thinking, 'My son does not respect me,' and that made you feel angry and upset."

It is helpful to physically draw arrows between different areas of the CBM to highlight these links and tell the patient that you are doing so:

"I am going to draw an arrow between these two areas that you mentioned. Does that make sense?"

Indicate any vicious cycles to the patient, whilst pointing at the relevant sections of the chart:

"There seems to be a bit of a vicious cycle developing here. When you think negatively you tend to feel worse and then react by avoiding seeing people, which makes you feel even more isolated and depressed."

Try to finish with a synthesizing question, which asks the patient to review the information and consider the next steps:

"What do you make of this? Could you use this information to help you in any way?"

Finding links should not be to the detriment of developing rapport and empathic relationships with patients. Remember that the CBM can be used review and understand the patient's difficulties, *even without* identifying links or achieving any specific immediate outcomes.

Reminders: Making links

- Making links highlights the relationships between different aspects of the same problem and may suggest new ways to solve complex difficulties
- Making links can simply involve summarizing the information presented by the patient
- Remember to physically draw the links as arrows on the CBM chart
- Finish with a synthesizing question to encourage the patient to tie together the information themselves

Setting and reviewing homework

Carrying out 'homework' enables the patient to apply any new concepts learned from the CBM to their lives outside the surgery. Compliance with homework assignments is one of the best predictors of the outcome of standard CBT sessions. Homework plays a key role in empowering the patient to make changes in their own lives.

It is important to explain the rationale for homework in general as well to discuss the reasons for particular tasks.

> *"For this approach to actually make a difference to your life, it is really important for you to think about the information at home as well. After all, we only have such a short time during the consultation."*

Remember to check whether the patient has any objections to the term 'homework', which has rather authoritarian overtones reminiscent of school or teachers. Many patients find the term amusing but a few may find it patronizing or offensive. It is possible to choose another word, such as 'self-work' or 'personal development work'. It can be left open to the patient to choose the most appropriate term.

Homework tasks should be discussed and planned collaboratively by the GP and patient together.

> *"What kind of homework do you think might be useful to you?"*
>
> *"How could you use this information to make a difference to your life?"*
>
> *"Can you see any ways to break the vicious cycle we have identified? What do you need to do differently?"*

The GP can make gentle prompts or suggestions for homework tasks if the patient is unsure.

> *"One possibility might be for you to try… What do you think about this?"*

Homework should involve simple 'SMART' tasks (see *Box 5.2*) that are easily achievable by the patient.

Useful homework tasks may include:

- Taking away a copy of the information gathered so far in the CBM, to review and add to further

Is the homework task:

Specific: clear definition of what the patient is going to do?
Measurable: easy to measure if the goal has been achieved or not?
Achievable: practical and realistic for the patient to carry out?
Relevant: useful and helpful to overcome the patient's problem(s)?
Timed: clearly defined timescale for carrying out the task?

- Reading a self-help CBT book or leaflet relevant to the patient's specific difficulties
- Recording relevant information, such as by keeping a diary of thoughts and feelings in different situations
- Simple behavioural tasks such as increasing activity levels or graded exposure to some anxiety-provoking situations

It is useful to discuss the importance of any homework task and encourage the patient to commit to carrying out the task.

> "*How realistic do you think it is for you to carry this out? Are you willing to commit to doing the homework?*"

In order for both GP and patient to remember what the agreed homework was, it is crucial for both parties to have a *written copy* of the task(s).

> "*Let's make a note of what you plan to do, so that it is clear and neither of us will forget…*"

During any subsequent appointment, it is essential to review and discuss any previously set homework. Ideally, homework should be one of the *first* things to mention when seeing a patient. After spending time and effort on completing a homework task, it can be very de-motivating and frustrating for patients if the GP later forgets or ignores the assignment. It also sends the message that homework is not really necessary or important and discourages patients from attempting future tasks.

> "*I am so interested to hear about your homework. What happened … ?*"

> "*I would be really interested to hear your thoughts on the leaflet that you read… ?*"

Overcoming difficulties with homework

There are many reasons why a patient may not complete a homework task. It can be tempting to blame the patient and assume that they are lazy or disinterested. However, it is far more productive and helpful to explore the reasons behind their lack of compliance. This is a similar principle for patients who do not comply with *any* medical treatment (e.g. drug therapy).

Using the CBM to approach any difficulties with homework can help to build an understanding of the problems that the patient is facing in 'real life' and also helps to find ways to overcome them. For example, highly perfectionist or obsessional patients may become overwhelmed by the amount of effort they perceive would be necessary to produce 'perfect' homework. Patients with procrastination problems may not 'get around' to the homework.

Box 5.3:
Overcoming difficulties with homework

Reason for not complying with homework	Approach to resolving problem
Patient did not understand the *importance* of homework	Discuss why homework is important: *"Why might it be helpful to do this homework?"* Remind patient that homework: • Predicts likely benefit of CBT • Offers opportunity to try out ideas in 'real life' • Learning a new skill takes time, effort and practice • Ask parents whether they expect their children to do their homework. Why? What is the benefit of homework for children? Is there any crossover with this situation?
Patient did not understand what they were expected to do	Remember to *check the patient's understanding* of homework tasks: *"What are you planning to try this week for your homework?"*
Patient forgot to carry out the task	Make a *written record* of homework tasks (e.g. in a journal or notebook) Discuss other ways to prompt memory: *"What could you do differently that might help you remember next time?"*
Patient did not think homework was useful or relevant	Design all homework in collaboration with the patient: *"What homework might be useful for you to do at home to follow on from this appointment?"* Check understanding of the rationale for homework: *"Do you think this might be helpful for you? Why is that?"*
Lack of time or motivation to carry out the task (seeing homework as a lower priority than other issues)	Discuss whether the patient feels their problem is important enough at present to put time and effort into changing. Avoid judgemental attitudes: *"How important is it to you to improve your panic attacks?"*

continued

	Express empathy for about hard work required: *"It can be really tough to make these kinds of changes, especially when life is often stressful and busy."* Discuss as a question of priorities rather than simply time: *"Is making a change less important than other issues in your life? Would you find time to pick up the cheque if you won the lottery?"* Try to get explicit agreement and commitment to completing homework tasks
Task too difficult to carry out (e.g. too anxiety-provoking)	Avoid being over-ambitious in setting targets – ensure homework is easily achievable: *"How likely do you think you are to be able to do this?"* Build the patient's confidence in small steps Discuss possible barriers *before* any potentially difficult or anxiety-provoking task: *"What might get in the way or stop you from doing this? How could you get around that?"*

Case example 5.5: Setting homework

Let's return for a final time to the dialogue between John and his GP. John has returned to see his GP without having completed the agreed homework – to read through some information about CBT and anxiety:

GP So tell me, John, how did you find the homework we agreed on last time? [*Checks written notes*] It was to read through that leaflet on CBT, wasn't it? What did you think about it?

John Well… I didn't manage to read it.

GP Oh right. What got in the way of you doing it this week?

John I just couldn't find the time – I've been really busy at work.

GP I see. I know it can be really difficult when you have lots of different pressures to cope with. Tell me, how important is it to you to improve your anxiety and depression at the moment? Are you happy to continue as you are at present?

John Oh, it's really vital to change. I just don't want to feel like this any more.

GP Do you think it will be easy to change?

John [*Looks a little demoralized*] No, I find it all so difficult. But I don't want to feel like this forever. I'm not sure what to do.

continued

GP Have you ever learned anything complicated or difficult? Can you drive, for example?

John Yes, I do drive.

GP When you were learning to drive, were you able to jump straight into the car and drive perfectly, without any lessons or practice?

John No! I had to have quite a few driving lessons.

GP And what happened to your driving after taking the lessons?

John Well, it got better and eventually I passed my test.

GP But supposing you hadn't made time to go to driving lessons, do you think you would have improved your driving that way?

John No, I would have never got any better.

GP Can you see any similarity between learning to drive and trying to learn a new way to cope with your anxiety and depression?

John I suppose they are both very difficult to do but it is really important to keep practicing otherwise I will never get any better.

GP Yes, that seems very true to me too. And how does homework fit in with all this? What is the purpose of it?

John I can see it is a way to practice and to get over my anxiety. It really is important to me to get there, so perhaps I should try harder to make some time for myself.

Reminders: Setting and reviewing homework

- Homework is a key stage which transfers CBM principles into an individual patient's life
- Homework tasks may involve patients reflecting on key information or trying out new behaviours and approaches to difficulties
- Tasks must be simple and must be agreed collaboratively by GP and patient
- Always take a note of homework tasks and remember to discuss them during the next appointment

Chapter 6

Understanding 'heartsink' responses

- 'Heartsink' refers to a subjective, negative emotion or feeling within the clinician

- It can arise in response to particular patients, situations or even colleagues

- Heartsink responses are based on the *clinician's own internal reactions*, including underlying thoughts and beliefs about themselves and others

- Labelling *patients* as heartsink is derogatory and inaccurate

- The CBM offers a unique means of understanding and modifying the clinician's individual heartsink responses

Understanding Heartsink

What is heartsink?

'Heartsink' refers to the negative subjective feelings that may arise within health professionals in response to particular patients, situations or even colleagues. The emotions involved may vary from feeling low or depressed to feeling anxious, angry, frustrated or guilty.

When GPs are asked about patients with whom they are more likely to experience heartsink reactions, they describe a remarkably diverse range of patient types and situations (*Box 6.1*).

Box 6.1:
Patient groups commonly described as 'heartsink' (Steinmetz & Tabenkin, 2001)

- Violent, aggressive or verbally abusive patients
- Complaining, never satisfied
- Manipulative, lying
- Demanding
- Appearing to lack respect for doctor's knowledge/experience
- Impossible to help (says "yes, but..." to all suggestions)
- Litigious
- Angry with the doctor
- Failure to cooperate with recommended treatments or suggestions
- Unrealistic expectations from clinicians or the NHS
- Unresolved, repeated complaints or presentations ('frequent attenders')
- Multiple complaints – presenting with a 'shopping list'
- Patients with psychosomatic complaints – doctor perceives there to be no 'genuine' problem
- Complex or vague presentations, e.g. "everything hurts" or "tired all the time"
- Talkative, rambling – 'difficult historians'
- High levels of anxiety (especially health anxiety)
- Difficult psychiatric cases
- Drug addicts

GPs do not always experience heartsink reactions in the exact same situations. One GP may find it particularly difficult to deal with demanding, professional people who have fixed ideas about what treatment they expect. Another may struggle with depressed people or perhaps those patients who ignore medical advice about the management of chronic disease such as diabetes or hypertension.

The definition of heartsink, therefore, depends on the *response of the GP* to a particular patient or problem, rather than being an inherent characteristic of any particular patient. Labelling people as 'heartsink patients' is not only derogatory and likely to worsen the GP–patient relationship, but is also inaccurate. The principle underpinning the CBM is that *we are all responsible for our own feelings*. This is as true for health professionals as it is for patients. The unpleasant, negative feelings that characterize a heartsink response arise from a GP's *own* underlying thoughts and beliefs about themselves and others.

From Theory to Practice...	Read through the categories of patients that are commonly associated with heartsink reactions. Which *two* patient groups would you associate with your own, ***most negative***, heartsink responses?
	Discuss this with colleagues and compare your answers. Look for both similarities and differences between your experiences.
	How can you account for these differences? How could you use the CBM to help understand this?

Reminders: What is heartsink?

- Heartsink responses are unpleasant, negative feelings which arise within health professionals when faced by particular patients or situations
- The term 'heartsink patient' is derogatory, unhelpful and inaccurate
- The experience of heartsink varies between GPs; it arises in different circumstances, with different patients and for different reasons
- The development of a heartsink response depends on the GP's *own* underlying thoughts and beliefs about themselves, the patient and the situation

Who experiences heartsink?

Heartsink is a common experience amongst GPs and other health professionals in primary care, but the circumstances in which it arises and the degree to which it affects different individuals is highly varied. Certain factors are associated with the reporting of greater numbers of perceived 'heartsink patients' (*Box 6.2*).

Box 6.2:
Factors associated with GPs reporting greater numbers of 'heartsink patients' (Mathers, Jones & Hannay, 1995; Butler & Evans, 1999)

- Less experienced doctors
- Lack of training in communication skills
- Lower job satisfaction
- Greater perceived workload
- Lack of postgraduate qualifications
- Underlying personal emotional problems (e.g. depression or anxiety)

Certain personality traits may also increase the risk of experiencing heartsink (*Box 6.3*). Such traits can be viewed as a cluster of particular thoughts and beliefs held by a particular GP about themselves, others or the world, which make that individual more susceptible to experiencing a heartsink reaction when faced by certain patients.

Box 6.3:
Personality traits
and associated
beliefs likely to
increase
heartsink
experiences

- Highly critical, judgmental or intolerant character (of self or others)
  "Patients should only present with 'genuine' medical problems"
  "The only way to deal with these patients is not to listen and just get rid of them quickly..."
  "That patient is simply a hypochondriac, attention-seeker"

- High levels of personal anxiety (includes difficulties coping with uncertainty)
  "I always need to be 100% certain that I haven't missed anything serious before I can relax"
  "Making any kind of mistake is a major disaster"

- Being overly nice or needing to be constantly liked by other
  "My patients must all like me; otherwise I'm not being a good doctor"
  "Patients must be given as much time as they need"
  "I can't get her out of the room – she would think I am rude if I ask her to leave..."

- Defensive personality or difficulty coping with criticism
  "Others should never criticize me"
  "I must never be seen to be wrong"
  "Patients should only come to see me if they will follow my advice"

From Theory to Practice...

Reflect on the patients who are most likely to generate your own heartsink reactions:

- Can you identify any personality traits and associated clusters of beliefs, which might result in your responses?
- How are these beliefs *helpful* to you? How might they be *unhelpful* or result in heartsink reactions?

Reminders: Who gets heartsink?

■ Certain GPs are more likely to experience heartsink (e.g. those with less experience, lower job satisfaction or poor communication skills)
■ The clusters of beliefs associated with certain personality traits make some GPs more susceptible to heartsink reactions in specific circumstances

Taking responsibility for heartsink reactions

Working in general practice involves caring for a wide range of patients with varied health needs that span physical, psychological and social dimensions. Such patients have varied personalities, health beliefs, behaviours and ways of interacting with primary care services/practitioners. Such diversity means that a 'utopian' work environment where health professionals are rarely or never challenged by 'difficult' patients is unlikely to exist.

In order to change heartsink responses, it is necessary for GPs to take responsibility for their own feelings and reactions. When faced by heartsink reactions, GPs often focus on changing *the patient,* but this is frequently unsuccessful and frustrating.

Remember that, as health professionals, GPs possess only the power to alter their *own* reactions to patients. There is no way to directly change patients. But by changing their own unhelpful thoughts or behaviour, GPs may be able to exert a secondary effect on patients by influencing the *interaction* or *relationship* between GP and patient (*Figure 6.1*).

Figure 6.1:
Relationship between
GP and patient

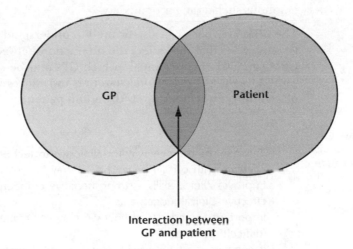

**Interaction between
GP and patient**

It is helpful to avoid thoughts that *label* and *blame patients* for heartsink reactions, such as:

> "*She was a heartsink patient who was overly demanding.*"

Instead, it is more helpful to focus on identifying a GP's *own* feelings and thoughts that account for the negative reaction:

> "*I felt angry and irritated because I was thinking that the patient did not listen to my advice and did not respect my knowledge or skill as a doctor.*"

By identifying a GP's own *individual* heartsink reactions, it becomes possible to identify ways to make useful changes or improvements to the situation. This may alleviate the sense of heartsink and improve skills for coping with the complex and difficult problems that GPs face on a daily basis.

Reminders: Taking responsibility for heartsink reactions

■ General practice involves caring for a wide range of patients, some of whom may be associated with heartsink reactions in certain GPs
■ Attempting to resolve heartsink reactions by changing patients may be frustrating and unhelpful
■ GPs only have the power to change their *own reactions,* which may have a secondary effect on the patient via the doctor–patient relationship
■ To change heartsink reactions, GPs must take responsibility for their own thoughts and feelings and avoid blaming or labelling patients

The CBM approach to heartsink

Using the CBM to understand heartsink reactions provides a useful approach to understanding and managing the GP's own, individual responses to difficult situations or patients.

The aim is not to eliminate negative thoughts or feelings about individual patients entirely, but to learn to manage these reactions more effectively. This helps to ensure that caring for certain patients does not exert an undue, emotional toll. It can also improve the clinical management of certain patients, which may be adversely affected by a GP's negative emotions such as anger or anxiety.

The CBM approach can also be used to understand patients. By identifying vicious cycles that may affect the interaction between GP and patient, the CBM can also discover ways in which GPs may be *contributing* to problems with 'difficult' patients. Understanding and addressing such difficulties will often improve relationships with certain patients.

Box 6.4:
Benefits of the CBM approach to heartsink reactions

- This may be the *only* way for clinicians to feel better and improve relations with certain patients who may be unlikely to change
- Improves clinical skills – strong negative emotion unlikely to promote effective clinical judgements
- Important to understand how we may *contribute* to problems with 'difficult' patients
- If negative reactions persist or get out of control, then GPs are at risk of stress, burnout or depression

Working through the CBM for heartsink reactions

Feelings associated with heartsink

Common feelings or emotions that arise during heartsink reactions include guilt, anger, frustration, irritation, anxiety, sadness or depression. It is important to identify which feelings are most prominent (*Box 6.5*).

Perceiving increasing numbers of 'heartsink patients' can also be a sign of a more serious underlying emotional disorder, such as anxiety or depression, which make it more difficult for the GP to cope with work-related

Box 6.5:
Identifying feelings in heartsink responses

- *"What does heartsink mean for me in this particular situation?"*
- *"What are the strongest feelings or emotions that arise in relation to this situation/patient?"*
- *"Am I experiencing difficult emotions more than usual at present? Do I have underlying feelings of anxiety, depression or anger?"*

pressures. In this case, it is important to address the underlying anxiety or depression directly.

Thoughts

The next step is to identify the thoughts and beliefs that underpin the negative feelings associated with heartsink reactions. These thoughts can then be *evaluated*, to decide whether they are realistic or helpful ways of viewing the situation (*Box 6.6*).

Box 6.6: Questions to identify key negative automatic thoughts

- *"What goes through my mind when I am faced by this patient?"*
- *"What is the worst bit about this? What is it about the situation or patient that provokes my heartsink feelings of [anxiety, anger, sadness...]?"*
- *"How do I see myself, my behaviour or my performance?"*
- *"What does the situation say about me as a doctor or as a person?"*
- *"Am I concerned that something might happen? What would be the worst thing?"*
- *"What do I think the patient thought or felt about me in that situation? What does that mean to me?"*

Behaviour

Understanding and changing unhelpful behavioural reactions can be one of the most effective methods of improving heartsink experiences. It is important to identify the behaviour itself, the underlying thoughts or beliefs which 'drive' the behaviour and the short- and long-term impact or result of the behaviour, both on the individual GP and others (including patients, colleagues and family/friends).

Box 6.7: Identifying and understanding behavioural reactions

- Identifying helpful and unhelpful behaviour:
  "How do I react to this patient? Do I behave differently with them than others?"
  "What happens when I feel [angry, anxious, low...]? What do I do differently?"
  "Do I know anyone else who might react differently? What would they do?"
- Understanding the thoughts/beliefs which drive the behaviour:
  "What makes me react that way? What might happen if I didn't?"
- Exploring the impact of the behaviour:
  "How does this behaviour affect me or others (patients, colleagues, family, friends...)?"
  "What are the likely short-term and long-term effects of this behaviour?"

Physical symptoms

Physical symptoms such as headaches, neck and back pain, tiredness, lethargy, abdominal and anxiety-related symptoms may be associated with heartsink responses. Existing physical problems may also be worsened by the stress, anxiety and low mood associated with heartsink. It is useful to identify the impact of these physical reactions upon the GP's daily life.

> • *"Am I experiencing any particular physical reactions when I feel particularly [low, angry, anxious…]?"*
> • *"What is the impact of these symptoms on me (at work, home, during leisure activities etc.)?"*

Environmental factors

Environmental factors may also have an important role in the development of heartsink. This might include work problems and personal difficulties, including life events or other life stresses. These can cause emotional distress, which may impact upon a GP's reactions at work.

A GP's own personal experiences of illness may alter their perceptions of patients. A GP who develops breast cancer or becomes severely depressed may later become more sympathetic to the difficulties of being a patient. Alternatively, another GP with a seriously ill child may become increasingly intolerant of a patient that she perceives to be a 'demanding hypochondriac', who takes up a large amount of time.

Making changes in certain environmental factors can be an important means of managing negative emotional responses. For example, choosing to work in a GP practice with supportive or like-minded colleagues or reducing the numbers of hours worked may improve job satisfaction and reduce the frequency of heartsink responses.

However, for a variety of reasons, it may be difficult or impossible to change certain environmental stresses. In this case, it is necessary to learn more effective *coping strategies* to manage these difficulties.

> • *Are you satisfied with your job? What are the major difficulties?*
> • *Do you have enough support at work and at home?*
> • *Do you have someone to discuss problems with?*
> • *Are you maintaining a healthy work/life balance? Do you participate in enjoyable activities outside work?*
> • *Do you have a 'healthy lifestyle' (regular exercise, healthy eating habits etc.)?*
> • *Are there problems with important personal relationships (family, friends)?*
> • *Are there demands at home (e.g. looking after children or family members)?*
> • *Are there other difficulties (e.g. financial problems, problems with home environment, ill-health etc.)?*
> • *Have you experienced/or are you about to experience any major life changes?*

Case example 6.1: Using the CBM in heartsink responses (I)

Dr T arrives for a busy morning surgery. She is 10 minutes late because of traffic delays and she already feels flustered and irritable. When she looks at her list of patients, she notices that Elizabeth is booked in for an appointment at 10 a.m.

Elizabeth is 50 years old and presents regularly to the surgery with multiple, changing symptoms. She has been investigated on many occasions, and has been diagnosed with non-organic chest pain, but has never been found to have any serious, organic disease. She is anxious and talkative and Dr T finds it difficult to know how to help her.

As soon as Dr T sees that Elizabeth is on her list, she experiences a heartsink response, with the following thoughts, feelings and behaviours:

Box 6.10: Dr T's CBM chart

Thoughts	Feelings
"Oh no, it's Elizabeth!" *"She will make me late for the rest of the surgery. The whole day is going to be a disaster now."* *"What does she want this time? There is nothing I can do to help this woman."* *"There's nothing wrong with her anyway! Seeing her is just wasting my time."* *"What if there is really something wrong with her this time and I miss it? I could make a major mistake and she would sue me!"* *"She blames me for not being able to cure her."* *"It is the patient's fault that I feel so stressed and fed up"*	Low mood Anxious and stressed Irritable and angry
Behaviour	**Physical symptoms/ biology**
Try to rush through the surgery Preoccupied by thoughts and worries about seeing Elizabeth When Elizabeth comes in, try to hurry through seeing her, e.g. not fully listening, poor eye contact, display less empathy than with other patients Quick to make a referral/do a test when she complains of a new symptom Focus on physical complaints	Headaches Neck pain Feels exhausted

Environmental factors/triggers

Difficulties juggling work and child-care arrangements
Elderly father has recently developed bowel cancer
In process of trying to sell house
Financial difficulties with current mortgage arrangements

Making Changes in Heartsink Responses

Evaluating thoughts and reframing unhelpful thinking

Once we have discovered the underlying thoughts and beliefs associated with our heartsink reactions, the next stage is to *evaluate* them, in order to identify and reframe any unhelpful or negative automatic thoughts and thinking styles (*Box 6.11*).

Box 6.11:
Checklist for evaluating unhelpful thoughts or beliefs

- What is the evidence for this thought/belief? Is there any evidence against it?
- Is this belief an 'unhelpful thinking style'?
- Is it logical or realistic? Is it fair? Is there another way to view the situation?
- Is it helping me to do my job?
- What are the pros and cons of thinking this way?
- What advice would I give to someone else in this situation?
- What is another way to view this situation that takes all of this new evidence into account?

'Evidence-based' or rational thinking

'Evidence-based' thinking is a rational approach to evaluating not only clinical decision-making, but also the way we interact with and understand others' behaviour. It avoids jumping to conclusions about others and counteracts the unhelpful thinking styles that represent distorted ways of looking at the world, worsening problems.

In order to practice evidence-based thinking, we must first be willing to accept that our initial outlook may not be entirely accurate, and that there may be another, more helpful perspective. This involves *thinking flexibly* and considering a variety of possible ways to view a 'difficult' patient, colleague or situation. We must then try to make a realistic evaluation of the situation – taking into account both negative and positive features, in order to reach a balanced conclusion.

Case example 6.2: Using the CBM in heartsink responses (II)

Let's return to the example from above of Dr T's feelings of heartsink associated with seeing her patient, Elizabeth.

Look again at the following thoughts. It is helpful to put a circle around one or two of *the most* powerful or distressing thoughts, which can be considered in more depth.

"Because I am running late in surgery, the rest of the day will be a disaster as well."

"There's nothing wrong with her anyway! Seeing her is just wasting my time."

"I should be able to help her, otherwise I've failed. If I can't make patients better I'm not a good doctor."

"There is nothing I can do to help this woman."

"What if there is really something wrong with her this time and I miss it? I could make a major mistake and she would sue me!"

"The patient blames me for not being able to cure her."

"It's the patient's fault I feel so stressed and fed up."

Using the checklist from *Box 6.10*, it is possible to test out and evaluate the most powerful or emotionally-laden, 'hot' thoughts:

Box 6.12: Evaluating Dr T's 'hot' thought

Thought being tested: *"She doesn't have anything wrong with her anyway! Seeing her is a waste of my time."*

Feelings associated with this thought: Anger, frustration

What is the evidence for this thought/belief?	*"She doesn't have any evidence of a serious underlying medical condition."* *"She comes in every one to two weeks."* *"The surgery is very busy and short of appointments."*
Is there any evidence against it?	*"Every patient that I see may have an underlying medical problem."* *"Even if it is not a 'serious' medical problem, she is still suffering from excessive anxiety about health, which may be as debilitating as a chronic disease."* *"Working in primary care means offering support to a whole variety of patients and problems, not just physical disorders."*
Is this belief an 'unhelpful thinking style'?	*"It is black-and-white/all-or-nothing thinking."*
What are the pros and cons of thinking this way?	Pros: *"Important to keep appointments free for other patients who may need them."* Cons: *"Makes me feel frustrated and irritable."*
Is it logical or realistic? Is it fair? Is there another way to view the situation?	*"She is experiencing genuine physical symptoms which she is terrified of – trying to understand her perspective may help me to feel less frustrated and annoyed."*
Is it helping me to do my job?	*"Getting annoyed doesn't help me deal with her very effectively."*

continued

What advice would I give to someone else in this situation?	"To try to address her anxiety to see if that helps her and reduces her attendances at the surgery." "Try to plan appointments in advance and be clear about time restrictions for 10-minute appointments."
What is another way to view this situation that takes all of this new evidence into account?	"Whether I like it or not, seeing patients like Elizabeth is part of my clinical workload, and getting angry does not help me do this effectively." "I would prefer her not to come in so often – this is an important issue for the surgery which I need to address with Elizabeth."

Now look at some of the other thoughts expressed by Dr T (above):

- *Which unhelpful thinking styles are represented by these thoughts?*
- *What feelings or emotions are likely to arise in Dr T in response to each of these thoughts?*

Try to identify some more helpful and balanced alternatives to replace Dr T's unhelpful thoughts.

The following table includes some suggestions for an alternative, more balanced thoughts and approaches to the situation:

Box 6.13: Balanced perspectives for Dr T's unhelpful thoughts

Thought	Possible associated feelings	Unhelpful thinking style	More helpful/balanced alternative thoughts
"Because I am running late in surgery, the rest of the day will be a disaster as well."	Anxious Fed up	Fortune telling (negative view of future)	"I *am* running late, which is stressful and frustrating. But, thinking how everything else will be a disaster just makes me feel even *worse!*" "It is not possible to predict what will happen later today but it may not be all bad! Anyway, I have survived busy days before – it's not a *complete disaster.*"
"I should be able to help her, otherwise I've failed. If I can't make patients better I'm not a good doctor."	Anxious Low	Black-and-white thinking Ignoring the positives	"There is lots of evidence that I am a 'good enough' doctor. No one can be perfect! I have good relationships with many patients and with colleagues. It is not possible to 'cure' everyone – that doesn't mean I am a bad doctor. Lots of people would find this patient difficult to cope with just like I do."

continued

Box 6.13: *continued*

Thought	Possible associated feelings	Unhelpful thinking style	More helpful/balanced alternative thoughts
"There is nothing I can do to help this woman."	Despondent Low	Black-and-white thinking	*"I may not be able to cure this woman's symptoms but I may be able to help her learn to cope better with them. At the very least I can offer empathy and support."*
"What if there is really something wrong with her this time? I could make a major mistake and she would sue me!"	Anxiety	'What if...?' statements Catastrophic thinking	*"It is possible that Elizabeth does have something genuinely wrong. This is true for every patient I see."* *"However, worrying about it does not help me find out. No one can be 100% certain – I just have to make the best judgement I can."*
"The patient blames me for not being able to cure her."	Guilt Hurt Anger	Mind-reading Taking excessive personal responsibility	*"She does feel angry and frustrated but she doesn't necessarily think it is entirely my fault. She knows I am trying hard to help her. If she didn't think I could help, she probably wouldn't come back to see me!"* *"She is struggling to cope with her difficulties and this makes her feel anxious and angry. It is not just a personal attack on me."*
"It's the patient's fault I feel so stressed and fed up."	Irritability Anger	Blaming others	*"Elizabeth is demanding and difficult, but **how I feel depends on my own expectations of myself and others**."* *"Blaming the patient for my stress will worsen my relationship with her and make me feel worse whenever I see her. I can't control how she behaves but I can control how I feel. Maybe I just need to accept that she is a difficult person and worry less about it!"*

Developing helpful thoughts and approaches to heartsink

Some beliefs, attitudes and thinking styles can *protect* clinicians from developing overpowering or overly frequent heartsink responses. These are summarized in *Box 6.14*.

Box 6.14:
Cognitive
factors for
managing
heartsink
reactions

- Rational, evidence-based thinking styles
- Increased tolerance and patience (acceptance of imperfection in self and others)
- Ability to manage uncertainty
- Learning to make compromises when appropriate
- Being flexible enough to change and learn from patients
- Maintaining a sense of humour (requires a flexible approach to the situation)
- Reduced need to *always be liked* – acceptance that sometimes others may be frustrated or that we may not like or be liked by everyone
- Focus on long-term as well as short-term goals (e.g. building long-term relationships with patients)

Building acceptance

'Acceptance' is an important concept, which includes the realization that humans are *flawed and fallible* and that we all possess both positive and negative qualities – nobody is perfect! This helps to avoid unrealistic expectations about both ourselves and others.

For example, by relaxing rigid ideas and rules about how patients 'should' behave or what constitutes 'genuine' reasons for attending the surgery, GPs may be able to reduce the level and frequency of heartsink experiences when these rules are (inevitably) violated by certain patients.

> *"I used to feel annoyed and irritated and give patients a hard time when they came into the surgery with minor illnesses such as colds or flu. I thought, 'They shouldn't bother me with such minor problems, it's a complete waste of my time.' But I realized that this was actually making me feel more tense and uptight – it was just adding to my stress.*
>
> *Now I try to stay calm and be more patient, by thinking, 'I know I see this as minor but the patient believes this is a genuine reason for coming here.' Trying to understand the patient's perspective and beliefs about the problem is also very helpful. I found that listening more to the patient actually helps me to educate them about their illness and encourage them not to come in for viral illnesses. They seem to respond better when I am calm and have taken their perspective into account."*

Developing patience and tolerance

Developing patience and tolerance can help to reduce feelings of anger or frustration when faced by people who do not behave as we would ideally like. Gaining a better understanding of the other person's perspective (*cognitive empathy*) is a useful way to make sense of other people's behaviour and is often helpful in alleviating feelings of anger or irritation.

> *"I used to be much more tough and uncompromising with patients. I was mainly interested in the medical side and was less open to other aspects of problems. Using*

the CBM has helped me to become more open and tolerant. I have more empathy for patients – and I find this helps me a lot as well as the patient."

Being 'good enough'

It is important for GPs to apply patience and tolerance to themselves as well as others. Being 'good enough' is a key concept for building self-esteem and is highly applicable for many medical practitioners, who often hold perfectionist beliefs and have great difficulty coping with perceived 'failure'.

"I used to be a real perfectionist and was very hard on myself if even minor problems occurred. I would feel really upset and annoyed with myself if I believed a patient thought badly of me in some way. Now I try to keep a more balanced perspective and remember that I have good relationships with most patients, but it is not possible to do everything for everybody. This helps me cope when things run less smoothly."

From Theory to Practice...	Do you ever experience heartsink responses which may be related to black-and-white thinking, a lack of acceptance or perfectionist beliefs? What thoughts underpin your responses? How could you view things differently?

Putting heartsink experiences into perspective

During heartsink responses, it is common for health professionals to over-estimate the importance or difficulty of the situation. It is often helpful to try to put things into perspective, by considering whether the situation is really as bad as it seems or whether, in fact, things might be a lot worse!

Case example 6.3: Putting heartsink experiences into context

Dr R has become increasingly frustrated with one of his patients, Roger. Roger is 62 and suffers from osteoarthritis of the hips and knees which causes him a great deal of discomfort and limits his ability to walk. He is also hypertensive and overweight.

Roger frequently attends the surgery but rarely listens to his GP's advice. Roger responds with "Yes, but..." to nearly every suggestion made by Dr R. He says that he can't lose weight and complains of side effects to most prescribed medication.

Whenever Dr R notices that Roger is on his list, he begins to feel anxious, agitated and thinks, *"This man is impossible to help. He doesn't listen to anything I say. I can't stand listening to him complaining any more!"* This makes him irritable with Roger and has worsened their relationship still further.

In order to try and get some perspective on his difficulties with Roger, Dr R tries a humorous exercise where he imagines the worst possible behaviour that Roger might do in a consultation. For example, Roger might:

- Physically attack Dr R or the reception staff
- Throw Dr R's computer screen out of the window
- Urinate onto Dr R's clothes while being examined
- Throw his medication at other patients in the waiting room
- Vomit into Dr R's desk drawer whilst the doctor is out of the room

This exercise helped Dr R see Roger with more perspective – Roger is a difficult character to deal with, but his behaviour could be far worse!

It is also helpful for Dr R to look at his *own* underlying thoughts and beliefs which may account for his difficulty tolerating Roger's behaviour, such as: *"If patients don't follow my advice it means that they don't respect me."* This kind of belief can be tested out and evaluated using the 'testing thoughts' checklist (*Box 6.13*).

Managing uncertainty

Learning to manage uncertainty is an essential skill for all health professionals. This includes developing and maintaining our clinical knowledge and expertise, to ensure that we are genuinely competent medical practitioners. But while learning and development may increase clinicians' confidence in their medical abilities, many *highly competent* GPs still struggle to cope with anxiety associated with uncertainty in consultations.

Managing uncertainty involves accepting that we can *never* be 100% certain of anything in life. Good clinical care involves managing *probabilities* rather than certainties and involves making an accurate assessment of the situation. This includes assessing the likelihood of particular risks and behaving accordingly.

> *"I used to find it really difficult to cope with uncertainty. I would wake up in the night thinking about a particular patient or wondering whether I missed something. It got to the point where I was considering giving up general practice, as I found it so stressful.*
>
> *What has been helpful for me was to realize that I just can't control everything. I can do my best for a particular patient, but it is impossible to be 100% certain that nothing will ever go wrong. And worrying about these patients at night makes it harder for me to work effectively because I'm tired and stressed out.*
>
> *Of course one day something could go wrong, but that is true for any GP. It is better to deal with this only when it actually happens. By continually worrying, I am living through the worst possibilities even before anything bad happens."*

The CBM approach is useful for identifying unhelpful beliefs that underlie excessive anxiety about decision-making or uncertainty in primary care. These include taking too much personal responsibility for factors which may be outside our control, placing too much emphasis on the worst possible outcomes, or having impossibly high standards:

"I must always be 100% certain about the diagnosis before I can relax."

"Making any kind of mistake will lead to disaster."

"I am entirely responsible for my patients' health."

"I should never miss any diagnosis."

Reflective exercise 6.1

Addressing uncertainty

Choose one or more of the above beliefs that might be associated with difficulty managing uncertainty.

How could the belief(s) be evaluated and re-framed to become more realistic and helpful? Use the checklist in *Box 6.13* to help you complete this task

---

Case example 6.4: Coping with uncertainty

During evening surgery, Dr L sees a rather anxious mother with her 14-month old baby, Lucy, who has had a cold for about two days but continues to eat and drink. Dr L carries out a thorough examination and Lucy is alert, looks relatively well and has a temperature of 37.9°C. There is nothing to suggest that this is anything more than a viral illness and Dr L reassures Lucy's mother, whilst offering a safety net by suggesting that if things got worse that she should seek medical attention and reminding her of any 'danger' signs to look out for.

Lucy's mother remains extremely anxious that her daughter might be seriously ill. Her friend's child had developed meningitis last year. After a long discussion, she agrees to try regular paracetamol and to monitor her daughter closely.

However, after surgery, Dr L starts to worry about Lucy, thinking:

"What if it really is meningitis? Maybe I missed something."

"Her mother may not pick up on the danger signs. If she gets unwell later, it will all be my fault."

"The mother was anxious – she must have thought I am not competent."

How could these thoughts be re-framed or re-evaluated? What is a more helpful way to view the situation?

From Theory to Practice...	Do you hold any beliefs which might make it difficult to cope with uncertainty?
	Use an example of a concrete, specific situation that you found difficult in order to clearly identify these thoughts and beliefs.
	What is helpful about your belief? Is it also unhelpful in any way?
	Try re-evaluating and re-framing these beliefs to be more realistic and helpful

Reminders: Developing new cognitive perspectives to heartsink

■ Developing *acceptance* that the world, others and ourselves are not perfect may help to reduce some heartsink reactions
■ Increasing patience, tolerance and empathy for others may also be helpful
■ Being 'good enough' is an alternative to a GP's own perfectionist beliefs
■ Heartsink experiences can be put into perspective by thinking up examples of other possibilities which may be worse
■ Managing uncertainty involves accepting that we can never be 100% certain of anything in life

Identifying and changing unhelpful behaviour in heartsink

Changing unhelpful behaviour is an important way of breaking vicious cycles and making positive, real changes in heartsink situations. The first step is to identify our behaviour in response to our thoughts about a particular patient. Next, we assess the *impact* of this behaviour and evaluate whether it is helpful or unhelpful for achieving both long and short-term goals for GP and patient. Finally, we can identify alternative behavioural strategies, which represent more helpful ways to respond to any specific situation (*Box 6.15*).

It is possible to make key behavioural changes *even if* we still experience a heartsink response to a particular situation. It is not necessary to *feel better*

Box 6.15:
Strategies for changing behaviour

- Make behavioural changes *despite* negative thoughts or feelings
  "What is a more helpful way to behave in this situation? Can I try this even if I still experience negative thoughts or feelings?"

- Behave 'as if...'
  "How would I like to feel in this situation? How would I behave differently if I felt that way?"

- Modelling others
  "Do I know anyone else who might behave differently in this situation? What would they do? Is it possible for me to try this?"

Case example 6.5: Using the CBM in heartsink responses (III)

Let's return, one last time, to the example of Dr T and her patient Elizabeth:

Think about Dr T's behaviour:

- Trying to rush through the surgery in order to 'make up for lost time'
- Preoccupied by thoughts and worries about seeing Elizabeth
- Trying to hurry through seeing Elizabeth: poor eye contact, not listening, less empathic than usual, quick to do tests or refer Elizabeth onwards if she complains of a new symptom

The following table considers the impact might these behaviours have on the GP, the patient and the consultation process and identifies what kinds of behaviour might be more helpful:

Behaviour	Impact of behaviour on GP, patient and consultation	More helpful alternative behaviours
Trying to rush through the surgery to 'make up for lost time' Preoccupied by thoughts and worries about seeing Elizabeth during other consultations	↑ stress and anxiety for GP Time management may become worse Increased risk of clinical errors Worsens relationships with other patients: ↑ risk of complaints Become irritable with colleagues	Take a few minutes to calm down Accept that you may be a little later than planned or ideal Proceed through surgery at safe, manageable pace Put thoughts about Elizabeth aside – focus on the patient in front of you
Trying to hurry through seeing Elizabeth: Not listening closely, poor eye contact. Less empathic than usual.	Elizabeth assumes you haven't heard and *repeats information again* and/or quickly returns to surgery Elizabeth feels aggrieved – relationship deteriorates Risk missing genuinely important clinical condition GP and patient feel hopeless and helpless	Listen *more closely* and give full attention. Make patient aware you are interested and prepared to give them your time Try to engage the patient in trying to *help you* to help them
Over-investigation or unnecessary referrals to 'reduce anxiety' Focus on physical complaints	↑ Elizabeth's anxiety about their symptoms: "*The doctor must think it's serious...*" More likely to return for further tests/referral: "*I need tests whenever I get the pain...*" Elizabeth continues to ignore emotional/social aspects of her problems	Investigation and referrals *when clinically indicated* not to 'buy time' or 'reduce anxiety' Discuss Elizabeth's anxiety about symptoms as well as symptoms themselves Use CBM to link psychological and physical factors

before we *behave* in a more helpful way. The process of changing behaviour may itself lead to improvements in negative feelings and thoughts, which can not only improve a GP's subjective experiences, but also improve their relationships with patients.

Reminders: Changing unhelpful behaviour

■ Behavioural change is a key way to break vicious cycles in heartsink reactions and improve clinicians' subjective feelings as well as relationships with patients
■ Considering long and short-term goals for both clinician and patient is important for evaluating the most helpful behaviour for specific situations
■ Behaving *'as if'* we *feel* better or *think* differently can be a helpful approach to making changes in behaviour
■ Modelling others may be a useful way to identify useful behavioural strategies

Using the CBM for teaching, training and mentoring

The CBM approach can be used as an individual, self-reflective exercise or used with a trainer, mentor or other colleague. The method can be applied to understanding heartsink responses to particular patients, as well as to other situations, including work-related stresses and difficulties with colleagues.

Using a video to record consultations can be a very effective way of identifying thoughts or behaviour that we may be otherwise unaware of. When looking at particular 'stuck' points or 'heartsink moments' in the consultation, it can be useful to use a CBM chart to understand and record our own thoughts, feelings and behaviour at that moment.

Tips for using the CBM with colleagues:

1. *Don't assume you 'know how they feel' (use cognitive empathy)*

   As the mentor or trainer, if you have had a similar experience, you must avoid the temptation of assuming that you know how the 'learner' thinks or feels. Their reaction may be similar in some ways to your own, but is also likely to differ in other ways. Be genuinely interested in discovering the key thoughts, feelings and behaviour that comprise their unique, individual reaction to the problem.

2. *Don't get caught up in clinical details (keep focused)*

   Remember that the aim of the discussion is to identify why the interaction with that particular patient has resulted in a negative emotional experience (heartsink) in the learner, not to discuss the clinical details of the case. It is easy to slip into this type of discussion, which may also be useful, but does not fulfil the function of helping to understand the learner's own negative feelings.

3. *Write down key information*

   Use a blank CBM chart to write down the key information about thoughts, feelings and behaviours associated with heartsink reactions.

This helps the learner to distance themselves from the problem and encourages a more flexible view of the situation. It can be helpful for the learner to write on the chart themselves.

4. *Use specific and concrete examples*

   Ask for specific, recent examples of situations when the learner experienced a heartsink reaction. Find out exactly what the reaction consisted of and what thoughts underpinned it.

5. *Use collaboration and guided discovery*

   Use the four stages of guided discovery (*Box 6.16*) to encourage the learner to take responsibility for understanding their difficulties and finding appropriate, workable solutions. It is particularly important to handover responsibility for learning from the discussion using 'synthesizing' questions (see Chapter 5 for further details about guided discovery).

Box 6.16:
Using guided discovery in teaching and training

---

1. Ask informational questions
   Open questions which focus on *specific* areas of the problem:
   "Tell me about..."
   "Give me an example of a situation when you felt this way..."

2. Empathic listening
   Careful listening and expression of empathic statements based on any unpleasant or distressing thoughts and feelings:
   "It must be very difficult to feel that way..."

3. Summarizing
   Reflect back information as a cognitive-behavioural summary, which encourages the learner to consider the problem from a new perspective:
   "So, this is a patient who behaved in an angry, aggressive way. You started to feel annoyed yourself, because you were thinking, 'he doesn't respect me'. You reacted by becoming defensive and refusing to do what he asked."

4. 'Synthesizing' questions
   Ties together relevant information and encourages the learner to make sense of problems *themselves*:
   "What do you make of all this...?"
   "How could you take things forwards...?"
   "Can you see any other way to approach this situation...?"
   "What might you say to a colleague or friend in the same situation...?"

Case example 6.6: Using the CBM for training and teaching

The following example of a GP trainer and a registrar discussing a difficult patient case illustrates some of the key skills for using the CBM with colleagues. Try to identify the following processes:

- Cognitive empathy
- Using concrete and specific examples
- Collaboration and guided discovery (look for evidence of summarization and 'synthesizing' questions)

Trainer Ok, could you start by giving me a brief summary of the patient...?

Registrar Well, this is a 38-year old woman, who has come in several times with headaches. She has a stressful job in banking. The headaches are classic tension-type pain and she is otherwise well. But she comes in with all kinds of downloads from the internet about headaches and asking for a referral to a neurologist. She can be quite aggressive and demanding in her manner.

Trainer OK, you have previously told me that you found this lady 'difficult'. Can you think of a recent time when you saw her?

Registrar Yes, I saw her two days ago.

Trainer I'd like us to work through a CBM chart to try to understand your reaction a bit better. At what point in the consultation did you notice any negative feelings?

Registrar Oh, as soon as I saw she was on my list.

Trainer And how did you feel at that point?

Registrar I felt anxious and a bit low.

Trainer OK, perhaps you could write that down on the chart. Tell me, what was going through your mind that made you feel anxious?

Registrar I was thinking, 'Oh no, it's going to be another difficult consultation' and 'she will come in and make demands about what she wants me to do for her.'

Trainer What is the most difficult part about that for you? What does it mean to you if she does come in and make demands about what she wants you to do?

Registrar I suppose it means that she doesn't respect me as a doctor. She just sees me as a 'tool' to use to get what she wants.

Trainer And what would be the worst bit about that? What would that mean about you?

Registrar That I am no use to her – that my role is not important – or maybe that I am not important.

Trainer And how does that make you feel?

Registrar I suppose I feel a bit hurt, actually.

Trainer Yes, that makes sense. What you have said so far is that when you were about to see this lady, you started to think: 'Oh no, it's going to be another difficult consultation,' 'she will come in and make demands about what she wants me to do for her. She doesn't respect me as a doctor. She just sees me as a tool to use to get what she wants. And that means that my role is – or I am – not important.' And those thoughts make you feel anxious and a bit hurt. Is that right?

Registrar Yes, that's right.

Trainer And how do you behave when you see her? Do you behave differently with her to any other patients?

Registrar I think I am more defensive and I listen less to her point of view. I find myself in confrontation with her a lot more than other patients.

Trainer How do you respond to her demands?

Registrar Well, I usually comply with them in the end. I did refer her to the neurologist but I felt really annoyed about it.

Trainer OK, let's add that to the chart. What made you feel annoyed? What went through your mind then…?

Registrar I was thinking that I should stand my ground. Giving in to her means that I am letting her get away with making demands and, sort of, pushing me around.

Trainer Do you have any physical reaction to seeing her?

Registrar I always feel quite tense and I sometimes get a headache myself.

Trainer I see. Is there anything else going on at the moment which might affect all this?

Registrar Well, I am quite busy at the moment, trying to revise for my exams. I am also trying to video my consultations, which puts me under extra pressure to consult really well.

Trainer I see. Well, perhaps you could take a look at everything we have written down. Tell me, what do *you* make of all this now…?

Registrar I think maybe I am feeling worse than I need to about how she sees me. She can't think too badly of me or she wouldn't come and see me at all. And I can also see how my being defensive and listening less will make things worse.

Trainer Yes, that's very true. Now, I'd like you to choose *one* key thought to take a look at in more depth. Which one is the most important to start with?

Registrar I think that *'she doesn't respect me as a doctor.'*

Trainer OK, great. Now let's work through this chart for questioning the evidence for thoughts. Is it an unhelpful thinking style…? What evidence is there that this is true…? Is there any evidence that it is not accurate…?

Reminders: Using the CBM for teaching, training and mentoring

- Use cognitive empathy and be genuinely interested in discovering the *unique* aspects of the learner's heartsink reaction
- Avoid getting caught up with clinical details and ignoring the learner's internal reactions
- Use a written CBM chart to record information
- Use guided discovery to encourage the learner to take responsibility for understanding and finding solutions for their difficulties

Chapter 7

Coping with negative thoughts

- The way people think about events and the *meaning* they attribute to situations will affect how they feel and react in various circumstances

- Challenging and re-framing unhelpful thoughts is an important method of altering vicious cycles and improving mood

- Learning to think more flexibly, rationally and compassionately are all important ways to reduce emotional distress

- A variety of cognitive strategies can be used to manage negative thinking styles

- Written thought records provide a structured method of identifying and challenging unhelpful thoughts

How can changing thoughts help?

Finding new ways to view difficult situations by challenging or reframing negative thoughts can alter the vicious cycles that contribute to the development and maintenance of mood disorders and emotional distress.

Remember that *thoughts about the meaning of the event,* rather than the event itself, are responsible for the way people feel and react in various circumstances. This means that changing the way people think about a situation may reduce any associated negative feelings.

Events are not 'good' or 'bad' – it is the *meaning* we attach to them that results in particular emotional responses. Events are simply things that happen. How *we feel* depends on our particular view of the situation. This view may sometimes be inaccurate or ignore relevant information.

The tale of the Chinese farmer

> There is an old Chinese tale about a farmer whose horse ran away.
> "What terrible luck," said his neighbour.
> "Good luck, bad luck. Nobody knows for sure," said the farmer.
> A few days later, the horse returned, bringing with it five more beautiful horses from the wild.
> "What fantastic luck," said the neighbour.
> "Good luck, bad luck. Nobody knows for sure," said the farmer.
> The next day, the farmer's son fell and broke his leg when trying to break in the new horses.
> "What bad luck," said the neighbour.
> "Good luck, bad luck. Nobody knows for sure," said the farmer.
> The next week, the army came to the area, looking to recruit all young men to the armed forces. They came to the farm, but because the farmer's son had a broken leg, they passed by and he was allowed to remain with his father.
> "What good luck," said the neighbour.
> "Good luck, bad luck. Nobody knows for sure," said the farmer.

Evolutionary benefits of negative thinking

It can be helpful to explain to patients why humans are sometimes *biologically programmed* to think negatively. Assuming the worst in a situation may actually help with survival and have an evolutionary benefit (*Box 7.1*).

Identifying negative thoughts

A multitude of thoughts, images and memories pass through most people's minds in response to events. The first step is to identify these thoughts and beliefs about particular situations or problems. The aim is to identify the

Box 7.1:
Evolutionary
benefits of
thinking
negatively

Imagine a grazing animal, such as a rabbit, which constantly needs to keep a watchful eye for hungry predators, such as foxes or weasels. If that rabbit catches sight of any movement, it often reacts quickly by running to safety. However, that movement is not always from a predator; it might simply be the wind blowing some leaves or grass. This 'better safe than sorry' approach helps the rabbit keep safe – it is better to run unnecessarily than wait to get eaten! It is mirrored in the human tendency to jump to the worst conclusion in negative thoughts of both depression and anxiety. However, whilst useful for the rabbit's survival, this response is often unhelpful and out of proportion to the 'dangers' encountered in modern human society.

most relevant or 'hot' thought, which is usually associated with powerful feelings of emotional distress.

There are three key areas to cover when discussing thoughts and identifying 'hot' thoughts:

- How does the patient see themselves? What does the event or situation mean about them?
- How do they think others see them? What does this mean to them?
- What are the implications of the situation? What does it mean for the future?

Writing down thoughts

It is useful to write down the key thoughts that are identified. This makes thoughts seem more 'concrete' and easier to clarify. It helps the patient to view their thoughts from a more rational perspective and to consider alternative perspectives which may be more realistic or helpful.

A written 'thought record' provides a structured method of recording, identifying and challenging negative or unhelpful thoughts. Thoughts can also be recorded using a CBM chart or patients could use a diary to note down emotional, cognitive and behavioural aspects of difficult situations.

Trying *not* to think about things

Many people instinctively try to suppress or control unpleasant negative automatic thoughts by trying *not to think about them* (*Box 7.2*).

The pink elephant experiment illustrates that trying to ignore or suppress negative thoughts may paradoxically *increase* their power. The brain has difficulty processing this kind of negative command. In trying *not to* think something, the mind must first recall what the thought actually *is*. This means that the unpleasant thought or image is likely to flash into the mind, where it triggers distressing emotions.

Box 7.2: Pink elephant experiment

For the next 30 seconds, try as hard as you can *not to* think about a pink elephant.

What happened? Did you think about the pink elephant at all? Was this easy or did it take a lot of mental effort?

Many people find that trying *not to* think about the elephant actually makes them think about it *more*. Thoughts and images of the elephant often pop into the mind despite efforts to keep them out. It can take a great deal of mental effort to concentrate on something else.

What can be learned from this experiment in trying to reduce the power of unpleasant or negative thoughts?

Trying to ignore or suppress negative thoughts is not usually a helpful method of trying to alter cognitive factors in the CBM. It is often more helpful to accept that the thoughts are present and then look at ways to actively challenge or alter them.

If it is difficult to suppress a relatively innocuous image of a pink elephant, imagine how much more difficult it might be to suppress terrifying images that may be associated with anxiety or panic disorder, such as visualizing yourself collapsing onto the floor and dying from a heart attack.

Reminders: Trying *not to* think about things

- Trying to suppress or control unpleasant thoughts may paradoxically increase their power and trigger more distressing emotions
- It is often more effective to accept the presence of negative thoughts and then actively challenge and re-frame them

From Theory to Practice...

Anxious patients are particularly likely to attempt to suppress unpleasant or frightening thoughts.

Use the 'pink elephant' experiment to discuss the impact of this strategy.

What alternative approaches could the patient take to manage their thoughts?

Distraction

Distraction is a useful short-term method of managing unhelpful, negative thoughts by paying attention to something else. It is particularly helpful for anxiety disorders, and may also be useful for depression when people are becoming overwhelmed by large numbers of negative thoughts.

Distraction is not a long-term solution that challenges negative thoughts or helps patients think more rationally. However, it does offer a simple, rapid, 'first-aid' strategy to reduce the power of negative thinking. It acts by taking the patient's mind away from distressing or unhelpful thoughts. This can reduce powerful negative feelings to more manageable levels, when it becomes easier to see problems from a more rational perspective.

Distraction differs from attempting to simply suppress or ignore negative thoughts because it involves a *positive* rather than a *negative* command for the mind. It involves trying to actively engage in a particular activity, which has the additional benefit of taking the mind away from negative thoughts.

For distraction to be effective, the patient's mind needs to be fully engaged with the new activity. The best activities are those which require focus and concentration to carry out, but are not too complex or difficult. There are many possible distraction techniques which are suitable for different environments (e.g. at home, in public places or at work). It often takes trial and error to find out which activities are most effective and absorbing for a particular individual (*Box 7.3*).

Box 7.3: Useful distraction techniques

> **Engaging in an absorbing activity**
> - Simple activities such as crosswords, word-searches, jigsaws or puzzles
> - Raising activity levels: go for a walk, phone a friend, do household jobs
> - Carrying out mental arithmetic or sums
> - Copying or drawing a simple diagram or picture
>
> **Focusing on the external environment**
> - Counting objects, e.g. numbers of bricks in a wall, number of colours or hues in a picture, all the blue objects in the surrounding environment
> - Looking out of the window and mentally describing what you can see, hear, smell or feel
>
> **Mentally focusing on or imagining something** (this is often the most difficult technique, but is sometimes helpful if the patient is unable to use any 'props')
> - Imagining in detail a different environment, e.g. a beach, forest or city street, including sounds, smells, and sights
> - Imagining a particular object, e.g. a flower, shoe or animal

Difficulties with using distraction

In the face of powerful, distressing emotions, it can be difficult for patients to tear themselves away from their negative thoughts and actually *do* the distraction technique. It is often helpful to plan in advance specific techniques to use for particular difficult situations or emotional reactions. Encourage the patient to try out the technique, no matter how badly they feel, and then monitor what effect it had.

There is a risk that patients begin to use distraction as a 'safety behaviour' to avoid *ever* facing problems or overcoming negative thoughts and beliefs. In this case, distraction can be counterproductive and serve as an avoidance tactic. Encourage the patient to use distraction as only the *first step* in managing unpleasant thoughts and emotions. The next step is to face up to and make changes in negative thoughts.

From Theory to Practice...

Using distraction to manage anxiety and panic

If a patient seems particularly anxious during the consultation, ask them to rate their anxiety on a scale from 0 to 100 (where 0 is no anxiety at all and 100 is the most anxious or panicky they could possibly imagine). If the level of anxiety is high, use the opportunity to practice distraction techniques.

Tell the patient that you would like to teach them some techniques to reduce their anxiety.

Then ask the patient to describe an object in the room or out of the window. Encourage them to describe it in great detail. If necessary, you can prompt the patient with questions about colour, shape, size, smell etc. Try to ask questions that make the patient *think* about the object (e.g. *"What else could you use this for?"* or *"What might the person outside the window be doing or thinking about?"*)

After a period of 2–3 minutes, ask the patient to re-rate their level of anxiety. If it remains high, consider repeating the experiment with a different form of distraction. For example, draw a diagram such as a star or other geometrical figure on a piece of paper. Ask the patient to copy or draw around the diagram as neatly as possible. Encourage them to focus on copying it *precisely*.

For example:

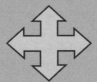 or

Once the patient's anxiety has decreased, take the opportunity to use this as a learning experience. Ask the patient:

"How do you feel now?"

"What do you make of the fact that you can feel so much better, so quickly, just by doing something else?"

"How could you use this information to help you in the future?"

"What was going through your mind that made you feel so anxious?"

"Do you see things any differently now you feel calmer?"

"What does this tell you about the way that you think when you are anxious? How realistic or accurate are the thoughts you have when you feel panicky?"

Reminders: Using distraction

- Distraction is a useful short-term strategy for taking the mind away from unhelpful thoughts by engaging with another activity
- It helps reduce the unpleasant feelings that arise in response to negative thoughts
- The most effective distraction require focus and concentration to carry out, but are not too complex or difficult (e.g. simple puzzles or mental exercises)
- Distraction can become unhelpful if patients use it to avoid *ever* facing difficult thoughts, feelings or problems

Broadening perspectives on difficult situations

When emotionally distressed, people often develop '*catastrophic thinking styles*', where they see things as more difficult or problematic than they really are. For example, they may overestimate the importance of an event such as making a small mistake.

It can be helpful to encourage the patient to put these difficult situations into perspective. How serious a mistake was it *really*? How important is this problem in *reality?*

One method of gaining perspective on problems is to ask patients to imagine how they might view the event in the future.

"*How will you feel about this in one year's time? Will it still be as important then?*"

"*How about in 5 years time? What about in 10 years...?*"

Another useful technique to gain perspective is to use a 'severity scale', where the patient rates different events on a scale, from extremely serious to unimportant:

Not _____ **Extremely**
serious   **serious**

This technique can help to gain perspective on problems by comparing them with other potential difficulties that could also arise. A range of possibilities, including serious events as well as more minor problems can be compared using the scale. These can be compared to the problem that the patient is actually facing (see Case example 7.1).

This technique is useful for challenging 'catastrophic thinking styles'. It does not suggest that the problem does not exist at all, but may show that it is not quite as catastrophic or devastating as previously thought. This may free up the patient to generate some useful solutions.

Case example 7.1: Using a 'severity scale' to gain perspective

Paula is a 35-year old secretary. As she arrives at the annual office party, she trips and falls over as soon whilst entering the room. She is not hurt and gets up quickly without causing any other damage. However, for a long time afterwards, Paula feels anxious and low. She even begins taking time off work to avoid facing her colleagues.

Thoughts:

"It was such a stupid thing to do."
"Everyone was laughing at me."
"They will all think that I am a complete fool."
"No one will respect me any more."

As a way of helping Paula to gain more perspective on the situation, her GP encourages her to look at a list of other mistakes that it is possible to make at an office party. They include some very unlikely or amusing possibilities:

Get angry and throw a drink over an important client
Make a scene and shout offensive comments at the boss
Smash a valuable antique vase
Get drunk and vomit onto the carpet
Get caught stealing money from colleagues
Start a fight and get arrested
Start a fire and burn the restaurant down

Paula's GP asks her to rate these possibilities into order of severity, using a 'severity scale'. Only after including all the other possibilities does Paula add the actual 'mistake' that she felt she had made onto the scale:

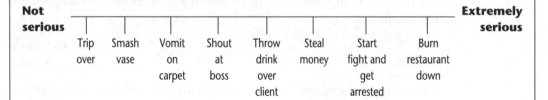

This exercise helps put the severity or importance of Paula's experience into perspective and helped to illustrate that her negative thoughts about tripping over were extreme and unfair.

Useful questions to encourage patients to learn from this exercise include:

"What do you make of this? How does it affect this major concern that you have about the mistake you made?"
"Does this give you any different perspective on what happened?"

From Theory to Practice...	If you notice yourself or a patient showing catastrophic thinking about minor difficulties (making a 'mountain out of a molehill'), try to put the situation in perspective by thinking up a range of other possibilities that might be *worse*.
	Make sure you include some amusing possibilities to keep the process light-hearted rather than critical.
	However, do not attempt this too early, whilst emotional levels are still very high. It is important to be empathic and supportive and take time to listen to the patient's (or your own) fears before trying to promote cognitive change.

Reminders: Broadening perspectives on difficult situations

- When emotionally distressed, people often view minor difficulties as a major catastrophe
- Asking patients to imagine how they might view difficult situations in 5 or 10 years' time can help to put it in perspective
- Using a 'severity scale' helps the patient to rate the importance of the event compared to other, more serious possibilities

Using pie charts to explore alternative perspectives

Pie charts can be a very useful tool for exploring a range of alternative explanations for events. The aim is to generate a more balanced view of events, by looking at a range of factors which may be involved. This can lessen the belief in any particularly negative or catastrophic outcome. They are useful in anxiety disorders, where people commonly overestimate the likelihood or danger of potential future events.

Pie charts can also be useful to challenge feelings of excessive responsibility or guilt after a difficult event.

Case example 7.2: Using a pie-chart to reduce feelings of guilt

Helen is a 45-year old woman who feels extremely guilty and low because her 16-year old son, John, recently failed several of his GCSE exams. She has become increasingly low and depressed, and has been sleeping badly. It has become difficult for her to think about anything else and she is not enjoying life.

Thoughts	Feelings
"It is my fault that John failed his exams."	Guilty
"I let him down."	Low
"I am a useless mother."	

continued

Helen's GP helps her to use a pie-chart to consider how responsible she is for John failing his exam.

GP Perhaps we could spend some time working out whether it really is entirely your fault that John failed his exams. It might help us to draw out a pie chart, where we make a list of *all* the people who have some responsibility for John failing his exam and give them each a slice of the pie. We will put you on the chart too, but not until right at the end. OK?

Helen I think so.

GP Hopefully it will become clearer as we go on. Let's start by making a list of *all* the people who had any responsibility for whether John passed his exam. Who else should be on this list?

Helen Well, I suppose John's dad.

GP Good. Anyone else?

Helen Maybe John's teachers.

GP Excellent. Who else?

Helen John himself.

GP And...?

Helen I can't think of anyone else.

GP Is there anyone else in the family who might have influenced John's exams?

Helen Well, yes, his grandparents do encourage him to work hard.

GP What about other people at school or friends?

Helen Yes, since he got in with a bad crowd, he has paid much less attention to his school work

GP OK great, now we have a list of people. Now, let's draw a pie chart and give a slice of the pie to each person. Remember, we are not going to add you onto the chart until right at the end. Let's start with John himself, how much of the pie should he have?

Helen Well, quite a bit I suppose, he is 16 now. About a quarter of it, maybe...

GP OK, that's true. Can you draw onto this chart how much you think he should have...? [*Helen marks on the chart a section of the 'pie' for John, himself.*] Now, what about John's dad...?

GP Now that we have finished the pie-chart, what do you think about the idea that it is entirely your fault that John failed his exam?

Helen Well, I can see that there are lots of people involved – it can't be all because of me. At the beginning, I felt like the whole pie belonged to me!

GP Yes, absolutely right. You do have some responsibility for John's exams – you are on the chart as well – but it is not down to you alone.

Helen I suppose that that however hard I try, I can't influence more than my own slice of the pie.

GP Exactly. How does that make you feel?

Helen I feel relieved and less guilty.

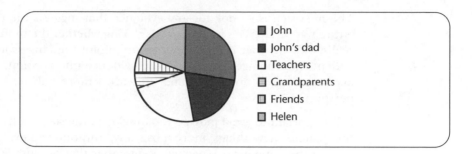

Reminders: Using responsibility pie charts

■ Pie charts can be useful to reduce excessive self-blame by helping to identify the full range of factors or people that may share responsibility for a particular event
■ They can also be used in anxiety disorders to explore the likelihood of a feared future problem

---

From Theory to Practice…	Do you ever feel anxious or blame yourself for events which may be outside your control?
	If you notice yourself or your patients doing so, try using a pie chart to share the responsibility more fairly.

Evaluating the evidence for negative, unhelpful thoughts

An important method of finding more balanced perspectives for difficult situations is to evaluate the underlying evidence for unhelpful, negative thoughts. This involves finding out the reasons *why* the patient holds a particular negative thought. People always have supporting reasons for their beliefs, which often seem very plausible and accurate to that individual. Without understanding these reasons, it is difficult to promote any cognitive change towards more helpful, less negative beliefs.

Box 7.4: Questions to evaluate the evidence for negative thoughts

- What is the evidence for this thought? What makes you think that way?
- Is there any evidence against this thought? Is there anything to suggest it might not be entirely accurate?
- Is it logical or realistic? Is it fair?
- Is the thought an 'unhelpful thinking style'?
- What are the advantages and disadvantages of thinking this way?
- What advice would you give to someone else in this situation?
- Is there another way to view the situation that takes all of this new evidence into account?

The next step is to look for any evidence that suggests the thought is *not* entirely accurate. This includes considering whether the thought is logical, realistic or whether it represents an unhelpful thinking style. Finally, the patient is encouraged to take all the evidence into account, both positive and negative, in order to come up with a more balanced and realistic perspective.

It is important to avoid moving too quickly to the stage of trying to 'make' the patient view things more positively, without exploring the *reasons* behind the patient's perspective. Remember that the aim is to develop a more balanced and realistic view of the situation, rather than just to 'look on the bright side'.

Case example 7.3: Evaluating the evidence for negative thoughts

Faith is a 44-year old woman who has been depressed for around six months. She has low self-esteem and is often self-critical.

Compare the following two examples of dialogue between Faith and her GP. Look carefully at the questions used by the GP and the response of the patient.

- How well does the GP explore Faith's *reasons* for her negative beliefs?
- How does the GP encourage Faith to change her negative thinking?
- How effective was this?
- How could the consultation be improved?

Consultation A:

Faith I feel like a total failure.
GP You say that you are a total failure. But is that really true?
Faith Well, I mess up most important things, anyway.
GP It is virtually impossible for anyone to mess *everything* up. I bet you did lots of things well this week.
Faith I can't think of anything.
GP Did you manage to go to work this week? How did you get on there?
Faith I did go to work and I just about managed to keep on top of my typing, but I keep getting distracted and making mistakes.
GP But you did go to work and did manage to keep on top of your typing? Surely this is of some value?
Faith Yes, I suppose so.
GP How about with your son? Did you care for him at all?
Faith Yes, I took him to school every day as usual and dropped him off at football training.
GP Did anyone else give you any praise or positive feedback this week?
Faith [*Sighs*] Not really. I suppose my husband did say he liked the lasagne I made.

GP It sounds like you have achieved all kinds of things this week. You took your son to school, went to work and made a good lasagne.
Would someone who was a 'complete failure' really manage all that?
Faith I guess not.
GP So how do you feel now?
Faith A bit better, I suppose.

In this example, the GP makes a good attempt to help Faith see her problems from a broader perspective, by encouraging her to look at the positive things that she had achieved during the week, instead of simply dwelling on negative events or perceived 'failures'.

However, there is little exploration of Faith's *reasons* for feeling low or for her belief that she is a "total failure". Without this initial exploration, it can be difficult to identify a more rational perspective that seems credible to the patient.

It is often more helpful to spend some time exploring the patient's negative belief and only afterwards to move on to looking for an alternative view.

Consultation B:

Faith I feel like a total failure.
GP That thought seems to make you feel very low.
Faith Yes, it does. I feel so terrible.
GP Tell me what you mean by being a "total failure"...?
Faith Well, I just can't seem to get anything right. I seem to mess up all the important things in my life.
GP What makes you say that? Can you give me an example...?
Faith Well, I am so worried about the effect of my depression on my son, Toby. I went to pick him up from school last week and I noticed that most of the other mothers looked so happy and normal. I am not like that and it has such an effect on Toby's happiness.
GP So you feel terrible because you believe that Toby is unhappy because of your depression? When you think about this, what goes through your mind? What does this mean about you?
Faith It means that I have let my family down. I am a failure as a mother. I should be making them happy, not miserable.
GP It seems like you are saying that you care about your family and want the best for them. So, when you noticed some other mothers looking happy, you started to think: "*I have let my family down*" and "*I am a failure as a mother.*" And, that makes you feel even more depressed and low. Is that right?
Faith Yes, that's exactly right.

This brief discussion between the GP and Faith helps to identify one of the major reasons that Faith sees herself as a "total failure". Now that this information has been identified, it may be helpful to move towards helping Faith to find ways to change this negative belief.

continued

Following on from the above consultation, how could the GP help Faith to develop a more positive or balanced view of herself? There are a variety of ways to approach this. What would you do?

The following dialogue illustrates one approach to this discussion:

GP Have you always thought this way?

Faith No, we used to be very happy, before I got depressed. But now, things have changed and however hard I try, it's not good enough.

GP I wonder if we could imagine for a moment what being a *total failure* as a mother would be like. It seems to me that must mean the mother wouldn't manage to do *anything* good at all. For example, a total failure might not manage to feed their children, wash their clothes or take them to school. Do you manage to do any of these things for Toby?

Faith Of course! I would never let him be hungry or dirty. I suppose I assumed that everyone does those things.

GP Do you ever hear any tragic stories about children who are not well cared for?

Faith Yes, you hear them on the news. It's really terrible that some kids are not properly looked after.

GP What other things do you do for Toby that might be important to his welfare?

Faith Well, I always make sure that he is well cared for. But I'm not sure if that is good enough.

GP It sounds like you are judging yourself very harshly. Would you think the same way if it was your best friend?

Faith [*Hesitates*] I suppose not.

GP What would you say to her?

Faith I would say that she did not choose to be depressed and that she is trying her best to cope with it. No one can be perfect.

GP That sounds like really good advice. How does all this fit with your idea that you are a "total failure" as a mother?

Faith I suppose that isn't really true. I do many things to care for Toby. But I still wish I could do more for him.

GP Did you behave differently with Toby before you got depressed?

Faith We used to laugh a lot more. I spent more time playing with him and helping with homework. We often used to go out at weekends.

GP Could you do any of these things even if you are depressed? This would mean behaving 'as if' you are no longer depressed.

Faith Well, I'm not sure. Everything is such a struggle and I don't have much energy.

GP Maybe trying to change everything at once would be quite difficult. Do you think there are any small things you could try?

Faith Well, I suppose I could try to help with his homework and play with him a bit more.

GP Do you think that might help you feel better? To try out some of the things you were doing before?

> **Faith** Yes, it might. But I'm not sure it would be enough.
> **GP** How could you find that out?
> **Faith** I suppose I could try it for a week or so.
> **GP** How will you check if these changes are making things any better...?
>
> In the above example, Faith and her GP discuss the *meaning* of being a "total failure" as a mother and begin the process of broadening her negative view of herself. Next, the GP encourages Faith to change her unhelpful behaviour. This is likely to support and reinforce Faith's more positive view of herself.

Using written thought records

Written thought records provide a structured approach to identifying and reframing negative thoughts and beliefs. Creating a thought record involves writing down information about the thoughts, feelings and behaviour associated with particular situations. The patient should write down how they thought and felt *at the time of the emotional* distress. In order to remember this information clearly, it is helpful to fill in a thought record as soon as possible after a difficult situation.

Regularly completing thought records will begin to improve patients' ability to think in more flexible and helpful ways and reduce unhelpful, distorted thinking styles. Eventually, automatic, balanced thoughts may begin to arise automatically in the mind, without the need for completing a written thought record. This may result in patients feeling less distressed in situations that would have previously triggered painful, negative feelings.

Using a thought record to identify patient's reactions

Learning to complete a thought record is a complex and sometimes difficult skill. It is often helpful for the health professional to work through the process with the patient. It is also possible for the patient to use CBT-based self-help literature to teach themselves how to use thought records (see Chapter 16 for suggested books/leaflets). In this case, the GP can take a supportive role in helping to overcome any difficulties that arise.

It is often helpful for the patient to learn to use a thought record in stages. Initially, it can be used as a type of diary, to record events that are associated with negative emotional responses. This involves writing down information about:

- Situation: what happened, where was it, who was involved? At what exact point did the patient begin to feel emotionally distressed?
- Feelings: Including the *severity* or *strength* of each feeling (rated 0–100)
- Thoughts and beliefs associated with the negative feelings
- The 'hot thought' (most powerful or relevant thought) (Greenberger & Padesky, 1995a)

Case example 7.4: Learning to use a thought record (I)

Sanjay is a 35-year old man who works as a planning officer for a local council. About three months ago he was promoted to a senior managerial position that involves giving presentations to other colleagues in the council. He has become increasingly anxious about public speaking and is beginning to avoid these situations, which makes it difficult for him to do his job.

He completes a thought record as follows:

Section of thought record	Useful questions	Possible answers by Sanjay
Situation	*"Describe a typical situation when you felt upset or emotional. At what point did you feel the worst? What were you doing?"*	*"On Thursday at 11 a.m. My boss came into my office and asked me to give a presentation about changes in local planning policy to the heads of department in the council."*
Feelings	*"Make a list of all your feelings or emotions. Rate how strong each feeling was from 0 – 100 (where 0 is no emotion and 100 is the strongest feeling you could ever imagine)."*	*"Anxious – 75, Tense – 70, Low – 60"*
Thoughts	*"What went through your mind that made you feel that way?"* *"What thoughts or images did you have?"* *"What is the worst bit about this situation?"* *"What does this situation say about you, your life or your future?"* *"Are you afraid that something might happen? What is this?"* *"What do you think that someone else might think or feel about you? What does this mean to you?"*	*"I'm not as experienced as many of the people in the audience."* *"I might get so nervous that I can't speak properly and won't be able to get my point across."* *"I don't have enough authority or experience and they won't respect me."* *"What if they don't agree with me or ask me questions that I can't answer?"* *"They will think I am foolish and incompetent."*
Find the hot thought	*"Which of these thoughts is the most upsetting?"*	***"They will think I am foolish and incompetent."***

Encourage patients to write down thoughts using their own words and in the first person (*"He thinks I'm boring"*). If the thought is a question (*"What if I say something stupid?"*) then it is also important to reframe that question as a statement (*"I will say something stupid"*). It is often also useful to include the most feared *answer* to the question, which underlies the patient's anxiety (*"If I say something stupid then others will reject me"*).

Choosing a hot thought involves identifying a key thought that is associated with the strongest negative feelings. It should not be simply factual, such as *"I did not enjoy the party"* or *"My son failed his exams."* Instead, try to explore and identify the *implications* or *meaning* of a particular statement, which is responsible for the negative emotion, such as *"Everyone thinks I am boring"* or *"I am a useless parent."*

Reminders: Identifying thoughts using a written thought record

■ Written thought records provide a structured approach to identifying and reframing negative thoughts and beliefs
■ Thought records can be used as a diary to keep track of difficult emotional events
■ Ensure that the thoughts identified include information about the negative *meaning* of the event for the individual patient
■ Patients can use CBT-based self-help literature to help them learn to use thought records

---

Challenging unhelpful thoughts using written thought records

Once the hot thought is identified, then it is possible to challenge its accuracy. Hot thoughts must be treated as hypotheses or guesses rather than definite facts.

Challenging unhelpful thoughts involves first gathering detailed information or 'evidence' that supports and explains why the patient holds this belief. Only then is it helpful to search for evidence that suggests the thought is not entirely accurate or fair. For example:

Thought:	*"I am boring."*
Evidence 'for' this belief:	*"I don't have much to say to people at work."*
Evidence 'against':	*"My friend Liz often calls me up for a chat and we have plenty to talk about."*

The final stage is to generate a new, more balanced thought to replace the original one. This takes into account the evidence both for and against the negative thought. For example:

"I am quiet in some situations but I have many friends who find me interesting and enjoy my company."

It is important that this alternative thought is backed up by genuine evidence from the patient's life, so that it seems believable and realistic. This process can be associated with a marked improvement in mood.

Case example 7.5: Learning to use thought records (II)

Let's return to Sanjay's thought record, about his anxiety relating to making presentations to colleagues:

Hot thought to test out:

"They will think I am incompetent and foolish."

Evidence *for* hot thought	Evidence *against* the hot thought
What makes you say that this thought is true? Has anything happened to prove it to you? Do any past experiences fit this belief?	Is there anything that shows this thought is not always true? Are there any times when you think differently to this? How? In 5 or 10 years from now, would you look back on this situation any differently? Are you ignoring any positives in the situation? Is this way of thinking an 'unhelpful thinking style'? What would be more realistic or helpful? If your best friend had this thought, what would you tell them?
"Many of the people in the audience have worked for the council a lot longer than I have." *"If I seem nervous then people will assume that it's because I don't have much knowledge."* *"Last week when I was talking to a colleague, he made a comment about how young I am."* *"In one of my previous presentations, I was asked a question that I could not answer and became very flustered."*	*"I have got the qualifications to do my job – that's why I was appointed."* *"My boss seems confident that I can do it – he could have asked someone else to do the presentation."* *"I may be less experienced overall but I have more training in my particular area than many others in the audience."* *"At the end of my last presentation, another colleague said it had been interesting."* *"I found out the solution to the question that I was unable to answer and spoke to that colleague after the meeting, who said he was pleased I made the effort to do so."* *"I have seen other presenters who were unable to answer one or two questions and no one thought they were incompetent."* *"There are many other aspects of my work that I do well. These things also affect how colleagues view me – It is not only related to giving presentations."*

Alternative/balanced thought to replace the hot thought:

Write an alternative or balanced thought which takes into account evidence for and against the hot thought. Try to be fair and realistic.

"I am qualified to give this presentation as I am more of an expert in planning than many others in

the council. It is not necessary to know the answer to every single question – I could look up the information afterwards if necessary."

Rate moods/emotions again

How do you feel now? Is it any different to before?
"Anxious – 40, Tense – 30, Low – 20."

Reminders: Broadening perspectives on difficult situations

■ Hot thoughts should be treated as theories or guesses and tested out by gathering evidence both 'for' and 'against' their accuracy
■ The next stage is to create an alternative, balanced thought, which takes into account both positive and negative factors
■ The alternative thought must seem credible and believable to produce an emotional shift

Overcoming difficulties with thought records

If, after completing a thought record, a patient does not feel an improvement in mood, it can be helpful to use the following checklist of questions:

• Was the situation that was described specific enough? Did the patient focus on the key moment of emotional change?

• Did the patient identify the 'hottest' thought? Are there other key thoughts that are generating the patient's negative feelings?

• Was the thought being tested directly related to the specific feeling that the patient was trying to improve?

• Did the patient write down enough evidence 'against' the hot thought? There should be more evidence against the thought than supporting it. Did the evidence 'against' the hot thought specifically include alternative ways to view any evidence 'for' the negative thought?

From Theory to Practice...	Pick a recent situation that caused you distress – it may be an encounter with a patient, a colleague or a personal situation.
	Work through the stages of the thought record by identifying any feelings and thoughts that arose
	Finish by identifying the hot thought that causes you the most emotional distress
	Next find the evidence both 'for' and 'against' your hot thought.
	What might be a more balanced, alternative view that takes all this evidence into account?
	Notice if you feel differently after completing the thought record. If not, use the checklist to identify what problems might have arisen.

- Does the balanced, alternative thought seem believable and realistic to the patient?
- Does the hot thought actually represent a core belief or a 'rule for living'? These are more deeply held beliefs which may not be effectively altered using a thought record (see Chapter 10).

Mindfulness

What is mindfulness?

Mindfulness is a form of self-awareness training that is based on the practice of meditation. It is not dependent on any particular system of belief or ideology. Mindfulness has been formally developed and evaluated as two practical techniques: mindfulness-based stress reduction (MBSR) (Kabat-Zinn, 1990) and mindfulness-based cognitive therapy (MBCT) (Segal *et al.*, 2001). There is increasing evidence that both approaches are beneficial in improving a variety of situations, including managing stress, anxiety, depression, chronic pain and improving coping with a variety of physical disorders (Kabat-Zinn *et al.*, 1986, 1992, 1998).

Mindfulness involves paying attention to the present moment. This involves observing our immediate experience, including any thoughts, emotions and physical sensations that may be present. Being mindful involves simply noticing these processes without trying to change them, either by attempting to cling onto enjoyable sensations or by trying to push away unpleasant or negative aspects of experience.

Reflective exercise 7.1

Breathing and mindfulness

It is important to *experience* this exercise for yourself – don't just *read* about it!

Sit for one minute and focus your entire attention on your breathing. Think of nothing else except noticing your breath flow in and out of your body.

What happened?

Most people find that their attention quickly wanders away from their breathing – it is very difficult to simply sit quietly and keep the mind focused.

What kinds of thoughts passed through your mind during this short time? Notice what a wide variety of thoughts you had. Perhaps you were thinking *"I'm hungry," "I've got so many things to do later," "This exercise is silly"* or maybe *"I wonder what's on TV tonight?"*

Did you get drawn into a 'chain of thoughts' about a particular situation? How long did it take before you noticed what was happening? Were you able to return your mind to the breathing or did you simply 'go with the flow' and continue to let your mind wander from thought to thought?

How much of life do we miss out on, because our attention is caught up with unproductive and unhelpful internal musing and loud mental chatter?

How can mindfulness help manage negative thoughts?

Our minds are constantly busy, generating thoughts, reflections and judgements about the world, remembering past events and planning or imagining future activities. However, we are often not consciously aware of these mental processes. This is like running on 'auto-pilot'. If we are unaware of the thoughts that are guiding and influencing our responses to events, then we limit our ability to cope with situations effectively.

Mindfulness represents the ability to stand back and become aware of internal processes and reactions, such as thoughts, emotions and physical sensations. It is like stepping back from a TV screen and reminding ourselves that, no matter how powerful and evocative the images are, it is just a film.

By simply observing thoughts from a distance, without immediately reacting to them, we may be able to choose to respond *mindfully* to a situation, rather than reacting automatically, according to an ingrained, often unhelpful, pattern of behaviour. In this way, mindfulness can reduce the effect of unhelpful thinking on people's lives and consequently reduce any associated negative emotions.

People may also react to negative thoughts and emotions by trying to push them away. This often creates a mental struggle, which may actually *increase* negative feelings such as anxiety and tension. In contrast, mindfulness creates a mental 'space', which can often help to calm an overactive mind, resulting in a sense of freedom and peacefulness.

Box 7.5: The 3-minute mindfulness exercise

> The following exercise is a simple and quick way to step out of 'auto-pilot' and connect with the present moment. Try it whenever you find yourself under pressure or in need of stress relief. Even a few seconds of mindfulness may help to manage stress and tension.
>
> - Sit upright in your chair. Close your eyes and ask yourself, *"What is going on inside me at the moment?"*
> - Notice whatever thoughts, feelings and physical sensations are present. Simply acknowledge and accept these, even if unpleasant, rather than trying to change them. It may be helpful to label difficult thoughts or emotions, e.g. *"Feeling anxious"* or *"Thinking about seeing Mrs Smith next week"*
> - Stay with your thoughts and emotions for a few moments and then gently bring your focus to your breathing. Follow each inhalation and exhalation as they flow rhythmically from one to the next. If your mind wanders, gently bring it back to your breathing as soon as you notice.
> - Finally, expand your awareness to include your entire body. Notice your posture, facial expression and any physical sensations present.
> - Now open your eyes. You may feel more settled and calm as you continue your day.

Developing mindfulness

The 3-minute mindfulness exercise is a good introduction to the practice of mindfulness (*Box 7.5*).

One of the key aspects of mindfulness is *acceptance*. This means taking time to become notice and acknowledge how we are feeling. Mindfulness also involves standing back from these reactions. As a result, although we may continue to experience unpleasant emotions or physical sensations such as pain or tinnitus, we are not entirely defined or enveloped within them. Instead, we become aware that there are also many other aspects of our experience which continue to exist despite the negative feelings.

Mindfulness is a practical skill, which takes time and practice to develop. However, the practice does not have to be complicated and there are many simple methods of bringing mindfulness into daily life (Box 7.6). Even spending just 30 seconds on practice can still be useful.

Box 7.6: Bringing mindfulness into everyday situations

> Most daily activities can be carried out mindfully, such as taking a shower or brushing your teeth. When you take a shower mindfully, try to be aware of the physical actions of rubbing soap into your body or shampoo into your hair. Notice the sensation of the water hitting your skin and how it changes as you move. Bring your awareness to how you are feeling emotionally – are you energetic, sleepy, unhappy or excited? What thoughts are associated with these feelings? Try to just notice the thoughts and feelings rather than getting caught up in them.
>
> Eating mindfully can be a surprisingly enjoyable experience. Try sitting quietly and maintaining awareness whilst you eat, rather than focusing on distractions such as talking, reading or watching TV. Notice what your food looks and smells like. Observe the physical sensations of biting, chewing and swallowing and notice the subtle variations in taste, texture and temperature of the food. If you get caught up in a chain of thoughts, simply bring your attention back to eating as soon as you notice.

Reminders: Mindfulness

- Mindfulness involves paying attention to the present moment and observing our immediate experience
- Mindfulness is a method of distancing ourselves from thoughts, which reduces the impact of unhelpful thinking and consequently reduces any associated negative emotions
- Becoming mindful of simple activities of daily life, such as eating or taking a shower is a simple way to bring the practice of mindfulness into daily life

Chapter 8

Changing unhelpful behaviour

- Changing unhelpful behaviour is one of the most important methods of breaking vicious cycles and making changes that have a genuine impact on daily life

- It is often easier to 'do something differently' than to 'think differently'

- Behavioural change promotes emotional learning ('in the heart') rather than simply intellectual learning ('in the head')

- Simple 'behavioural experiments' can easily be used with primary care patients

- Behavioural experiments are relevant for a wide variety of clinical problems, including managing chronic disease and emotional disorders

The importance of changing behaviour

Changing behaviour can be one of the most powerful methods of testing and changing negative or unhelpful thoughts or feelings. Testing out alternative, more balanced beliefs in daily life will make them seem more credible and believable to the patient. Whilst thinking and talking about issues can be helpful, often the best way to prove something is to try it out by behaving differently.

Behavioural change is so effective because it provides powerful *evidence* for changes in thoughts or feelings. Techniques that focus directly on cognitive change and altering unhelpful thinking styles create a kind of 'intellectual' belief in the alternative, balanced thoughts. This is often described as believing with 'the head'. However, patients may still say "*I do know that I should think more rationally, but the negative thoughts still feel true.*" In comparison, the changes in belief that arise from making behavioural change take place on a more 'emotional' level, or 'in the heart'.

It is helpful to combine both cognitive and behavioural change. For example, the belief "*I am boring and people don't want to hear my views*" can be discussed and reframed on a verbal or intellectual basis, to a new, more balanced perspective such as, "*Many people do find my conversation interesting.*" However, without also changing the behaviour that is associated with the belief (e.g. avoiding social contact, making poor eye contact with others, not speaking in the company of others), the belief in the new perspective is likely to remain limited. By changing behaviour (e.g. acting 'as if' I am interesting, making eye contact and listening to others, and trying out making conversation), and noting the impact of the change, the patient gathers evidence to reinforce the new, more helpful belief ("*If I do talk to others then they often seem interested in what I have to say*").

Reminders: The importance of changing behaviour

- Changing behaviour is a powerful method of changing negative thoughts or feelings
- Trying new behaviour can often provide evidence for alternative, balanced beliefs that makes them seem more credible and believable
- Behaving 'as if' we hold more balanced or helpful beliefs can set up a 'positive cycle' which reinforces and promotes positive change

---

Involving patients in behavioural changes

Patients must be actively involved in the cognitive-behavioural approach and should be encouraged to take ownership for making behavioural changes. With this aim in mind, GPs must try to avoid making too many directive statements or suggestions for change.

Health professionals frequently offer advice or make suggestions that are inappropriate or impossible to apply within a patient's real-life situation. Then, when patients 'fail' to comply, the GP feels frustrated and the relationship may deteriorate. Most patients are more likely to follow through ideas they have generated themselves, rather than advice given by others.

'Yes, but...' responses are a common indicator that suggestions are too prescribed or directive. Patients may say this directly (e.g. *"Well, yes, I know I should exercise more, but I just don't have time"*) or, may outwardly agree, but simply ignore the suggestion once they leave the surgery. This lack of 'concordance' is often seen when prescribing medication.

To avoid 'Yes, but...' responses, the simple answer is for the GP to make fewer suggestions. Instead, *hand over responsibility to the patient* to generate their own suggestions and choices about realistic, appropriate or useful changes in behaviour.

> *"What do you think might help you in this situation...?"*
>
> *"You are an 'expert' in your own life. What do you think might work for you?"*
>
> *"What do you think you could do differently...?"*

From Theory to Practice...	Watch out for 'Yes, but...' responses to your suggestions.
	When you become aware of this, make an effort to *stop* making directive suggestions or giving advice.
	Instead, hand back responsibility to the patient.

Setting realistic expectations for improvement

The process of making behavioural changes should be broken up into small, manageable steps. These are easier to achieve and provide a building block for further change. Patients can be encouraged to carry out a variety of simple experiments to look at different aspects of their difficulties.

It may be important to remind patients that making change is not always easy. It is helpful to expect difficulties and to plan ways to actively face and overcome any problems that may arise, rather than simply giving up when things do not immediately go according to plan.

From Theory to Practice...	Encourage patients to have realistic expectations about their progress by drawing out a series of boxes, joined by arrows:

	Tell the patient that the box at the far left represents how they are at the current time – ask the patient to briefly describe what this means to them, e.g. *feeling very depressed, not going out, not working.*

From Theory to Practice... *continued*	The box at the far right represents where they would *like to get to*, e.g. *no longer depressed, back at work, good social life.*
	Next, ask the patient to imagine how they might feel in the series of boxes in between:
	still quite low, going out a little more but not really enjoying it, not yet back at work
	↓
	mood lifts at times, more active generally, thinking about work
	↓
	depression improving (still down occasionally), better social life, preparing to return to work
	This helps set realistic targets. It may also be helpful for the patient to realize that it is normal to continue to experience some unpleasant symptoms, even whilst life is improving.

Reminders: Setting realistic expectations for improvement

■ Break down behavioural changes into small steps which are easy to achieve and form building blocks for future change
■ Patients should carry out multiple, small experiments to investigate different aspects of problems
■ Patients should expect to experience problems and should be encouraged to actively look for ways to overcome them
■ Encourage patients to be realistic about expected progress with their difficulties

Making a cost–benefit analysis of behaviour

Carrying out a 'cost–benefit' analysis of a particular behaviour can be useful in motivating the patient to make behavioural changes. It can also help to identify the reasons why a patient may continue to behave in a seemingly destructive, negative or 'non-compliant' way.

Making a cost–benefit analysis is a relatively straightforward process, which involves creating a written list of the *advantages/benefits* and *disadvantages/ costs* of a particular behaviour. The patient can then be asked to reflect upon the information gathered. When the disadvantages for a particular behaviour outweigh the apparent advantages, the individual is likely to be more motivated to make change. It can also be useful to spend time discussing alternative, less problematic ways of achieving the advantages.

Case example 8.1: Cost–benefit analysis of taking medication for hypertension

Mohammed is a 64-year old man with hypertension – his last blood pressure reading was 165/101. He is also a smoker with no other cardio-vascular risk factors. He has been prescribed anti-hypertensive medication but his blood pressure remains consistently elevated. During one surgery visit, he admits to his GP that he only takes his medication intermittently. His GP suggests that Mohammed makes a cost–benefit analysis of this behaviour:

Behaviour: Missing doses of anti-hypertension medication

Advantages/benefits	Disadvantages/costs
"I don't like the unpleasant side effects of taking the tablets." *"Not taking it every day stops my body getting dependent on the medication."* *"I don't want my life to be ruled or controlled by having to take tablets every day."*	*"My blood pressure will stay high if I don't take medication regularly."* *"Having high blood pressure can increase my chances of getting seriously ill, like having a heart attack or a stroke."* *"It is important to me to remain as healthy as possible, for the sake of my wife and family."* *"Knowing my blood pressure is high makes me feel quite anxious."* *"I don't give my body a chance to get used to the medication – side effects may settle down or I may get more used to them."* *"I could switch medication if the side effects are unbearable."* *"The doctor says that these kind of tablets are not addictive."*

Alternative perspective: Taking my medication regularly might bring down my blood pressure and make me feel more in control of my health. It will also cut down my risk of getting seriously ill in the future.

How could I behave differently? Make a big effort to take my medication every day, as prescribed. I will come and see the doctor if the tablets do not agree with me.

From Theory to Practice...	Think about the different types of patient who might benefit from using a cost–benefit analysis of a particular behaviour. This might include unhelpful or 'unhealthy' behaviour such as smoking, over-eating, avoiding exercise or not taking medication.

From Theory to Practice... *continued*	Practice using a cost–benefit analysis yourself if you have any behaviour that you would like to change.
	Try using this approach with one or two patients. Remember to keep an open mind and remain interested in discovering the perceived benefits of the behaviour before moving to discussions about disadvantages or costs.

Reminders: Making a cost–benefit analysis of behaviour

■ Making a cost–benefit analysis can help to motivate the patient to make helpful changes in behaviour
■ Use the approach to explore the patient's underlying beliefs, which may help to explain seemingly destructive or unhelpful behaviour
■ This provides an opportunity to provide patients with useful information to help them make decisions about helpful future behaviour

Using 'behavioural experiments'

Behavioural experiments are specifically designed approaches to changing behaviour. There are three main purposes of behavioural experiments:

1. To demonstrate the principles of CBT for individual patients, by illustrating links between thoughts, feelings and behaviour (e.g. observing the impact of focusing on bodily symptoms in health anxiety)
2. To decrease the level of belief in negative, unhelpful thoughts and increase belief in alternative, more helpful thoughts
3. To alter the level of unpleasant emotion (e.g. using distraction)

Behavioural experiments allow people to test out negative beliefs or predictions and to construct and test out new, more adaptive perspectives. Provided the patient remains open to the possibility that an alternative belief *might* have some validity, it is not necessary for them to fully believe it in order to carry out an effective behavioural experiment. This approach is useful for 'yes, but...' responses. Instead of offering the answer, encourage the patient to *find out for themselves*, by testing out their belief in practice.

Behavioural experiments can be used to collect data that support the development of more positive or helpful beliefs. This is important if the patient simply does not have enough factual material to decide whether or not a particular negative thought is true. For example, people who suffer from social anxiety may hold a belief that "*It is abnormal to feel anxious when meeting others – it means there is something wrong with me.*" It is only by testing out this belief in practice, perhaps by conducting a small survey of other people's experiences, that patients are able to convincingly establish a new belief such as, "*It is common to feel anxious when meeting others.*"

Behavioural experiments can also be used to find methods of reducing unpleasant emotional experiences, such as by testing out the impact of using distraction techniques or of using gentle exercise to increase energy in depression.

Identifying relevant behavioural experiments

In order to be effective, behavioural experiments must be directly relevant to individual patients and should test out the specific negative, unhelpful beliefs that maintain their problems. It is therefore essential to spend some time developing a thorough understanding of the patient's problems using the CBM.

Behavioural experiments can be *active*, where the patient tries out something different and notes down the impact of the new behaviour. Other experiments may be simply *observational*. This might involve asking a patient to observe other people in order to identify new ways of behaving in target situations (which can later be tested out during a more active experiment). It may also be useful for patients to gather a range of information or opinions from other people about particular questions or concerns.

Reminders: Behavioural experiments

■ Behavioural experiments allow people to test out negative beliefs or predictions and to construct and test out new perspectives
■ The approach encourages the patient to *find out for themselves*, by testing out their specific negative beliefs in practice
■ Behavioural experiments can be used to collect data that supports more helpful beliefs or to find methods of reducing unpleasant emotional experiences
■ Experiments may be active, where the patient tries out something different, or may involve observing or asking the opinions of other people

Designing and implementing effective behavioural experiments

It is important to take a systematic approach to designing and implementing behavioural experiments. This maximizes the potential benefit for each individual patient (*Figures 8.1 and 8.2*).

Stages of designing behavioural experiments:

1. *Identify the problem*
   This involves identifying the patient's current behavioural strategies for dealing with their difficulties, as well as any relevant thoughts, fears or negative predictions about making change.

Figure 8.1:
Overview of
behavioural
experiments

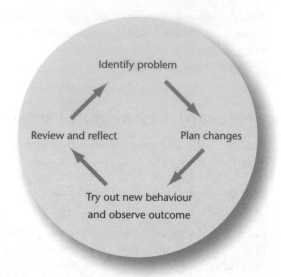

Identify problem

Review and reflect

Plan changes

Try out new behaviour
and observe outcome

Figure 8.2:
Behavioural
experiment
planning chart

Thought being tested:	
What am I going to do? (What, where, when...?)	
What do I predict will happen?	
What problems might arise with this plan?	
How could these problems be overcome?	
What happened when I tried the experiment?	

What have I learned from this experiment?

Box 8.1: Areas
to address when
planning
behavioural
experiments

- What specific thought(s) could be tested using behavioural experiments? Rate the current level of belief in these thoughts.
- Which negative emotions are these thoughts associated with?
- What unhelpful behaviours are currently maintaining the negative thoughts?
- What could be a more balanced or rational belief to test?
- How could these thoughts or predictions be tested in practice?
- What does the patient predict will happen if they change the behaviour?

It is necessary to identify the specific target thoughts to challenge with the experiment (e.g. in depression, *"I am too tired to do anything,"* *"Doing activities will make me feel worse"*).

It is important to be specific when identifying particular thoughts and negative predictions to test out. For example, a socially anxious patient may believe, *"I will look foolish in front of others,"* but this should be discussed in more depth to identify in what precise ways they fear 'looking foolish', such as *"I will babble uncontrollably"* or *"My mind will go blank and I will say nothing at all."*

The next stage is to identify which behaviours could be altered or 'manipulated' in order to challenge the underlying negative thoughts. It is often helpful to identify a specific, testable prediction based on the patient's thoughts. This involves identifying what the patient thinks will be the consequences of changing the behaviour.

Case example 8.2: Improving sleep patterns (I)

Trisha is 28 years old and has been depressed for over a year. She is a single mother with a 4-year old daughter. She feels constantly exhausted and lethargic, but sleeps poorly at night – she finds it difficult to drop off to sleep and tends to oversleep in the morning. She has begun taking daytime naps to try to compensate for this.

Her GP helps Trisha to plan out a behavioural experiment to test out the effect of changing her behaviour:

Key thought(s) to test:	*"I need to take naps to catch up on my lost sleep otherwise I can't cope during the day."* *"Taking naps makes me feel better when I'm down."*
What negative emotions are associated with these thought?	Lethargy, feeling down
What current behaviours are reinforcing negative thoughts?	Oversleeping in mornings may make sleep at night worse
What does the patient predict will happen?	*"I will feel more tired if I don't take a nap."* *"My mood will get worse if I'm more tired."*
What could be a more balanced and rational belief?	*"Taking naps makes me feel more tired and low."* *"If I stop taking naps, I will still be able to cope and will sleep better at night."*

---

2. *Plan behavioural changes*

The next stage is to decide what behaviour to change in order to test out the relevant thoughts. This involves working out a detailed plan of how to conduct the experiment, which includes anticipating and preparing for any difficulties that might arise.

Experiments should be planned as 'no lose' experiences. This means keeping a genuinely open mind about what might arise. Some apparently unrealistic negative thoughts may turn out to be true. However, discovering this is still useful, because it enables the patient to then focus on effective problem-solving to find a way to overcome it.

The experiments chosen should be relevant, realistic and acceptable to the patient but should not be overly complex or challenging. The GP must be supportive and openly acknowledge the difficulty of trying out something different. This helps the patient face potentially difficult or frightening situations.

Remember to convey enthusiasm and interest in the experiment and its results to the patient, which might encourage them to carry it out.

Box 8.2:
Checklist for planning behavioural changes

Planning what experiment to try
- How could you test out whether the key thought is true?
- What could you try doing differently?

Planning how to go about the experiment
- What are the details of the plan (what, when, where, who....)?
- How could we make this a 'no-lose' experiment?

Preparing for potential difficulties with the experiment
- Do you understand what you are trying to do and why?
- How likely are you to try it? Would anything make you more likely to do so?
- What problems might arise with trying this? How could you overcome these?

Case example 8.3: Improving sleep patterns (II)

Let's return to the example of Trisha, who has identified the following alternative thought to test out: "*If I stop taking naps, I will still be able to cope and will sleep better at night.*"

Trisha and her GP agree that a helpful way to test this thought would be to compare the two strategies (napping versus not napping) over a two-week period.

During the first week, Trisha planned not make any changes to her current sleep pattern, but would monitor how often she napped, how much sleep she got at night and how tired she felt during the day.

During the second week, she would try to avoid napping. She would continue to monitor her tiredness and sleep at night.

Potential difficulties were that she might feel so tired that she was unable to avoid dropping off to sleep. To try to overcome this problem, Trisha planned out some enjoyable or engaging activities to try at these times instead.

3. *Try out new behaviour and observe what happened*

The next step is for the patient to try out the new behaviour in practice. They should be encouraged to keep a written record of what they tried and what happened, in terms of changes in thoughts, feelings or physical symptoms. In some cases, it may also be necessary to note the reactions of other people.

Box 8.3:
Checklist for assessing the outcome of making behavioural changes

- What did you actually do? Was this what you had planned? If not, what got in the way?
- What thoughts arose in your mind before, during and after the experiment?
- How did you *feel*, before, during and after the experiment?
- Did you experience any changes in physical symptoms?
- What did you notice about other people's reactions?

Case example 8.4: Improving sleep patterns (III)

Trisha returned to visit her GP three weeks after the experiment had been carried out.

She found that it had been difficult to reduce her daytime naps, but she had successfully managed to reduce the number of naps from 11 in the first week down to 3 in the second week.

She noticed that at the start of the week it was more difficult to avoid napping and she did feel more tired, but she had still managed to cope with daily life. By the end of the week, she found it easier and felt less lethargic and tired than previously. She also noticed that she was sleeping better at night and that her overall mood had improved.

4. *Review and reflection*

The final stage is for patients to review the results of the experiment and reflect on what it means for them. This is essential for making sense of the information and learning from the experiment.

It is also important to reflect on any difficulties that arose with carrying out the experiment and look for ways to move forwards using this information. This may mean trying another experiment to test out another relevant belief. Sometimes patients may try a behaviour which does not help them or a feared prediction may come true. In this case, it is important to encourage patients to creatively *problem-solve* rather than just give up entirely.

Box 8.4:
Questions for
reviewing and
reflecting on
behavioural
experiments

Learning from the experience
- What do you make of what you found?
- Does the information alter your view of your original, negative thought or prediction?
- Does it add any support to your new, alternative thought?
- Did you discover anything else?
- How could you apply this knowledge to improve things for you on a day-to-day basis?

Making future progress and overcoming problems
- Do you have any continuing doubts? How could you test these?
- Are there any other relevant thoughts which may need to test out?
- If things did not turn out as you had expected or hoped, how could you overcome these difficulties in future?
- What can you do next to continue to make progress?

Case example 8.5: Improving sleep patterns (IV)

Trisha concluded that she could cope without napping and that this did improve her night-time sleep, which made her less tired overall. She had also found that, by increasing activity instead of napping, she had managed to achieve more during her day, which gave her an increased sense of satisfaction.

More case examples of behavioural experiments

Case example 8.6: Overcoming procrastination

Keith is a journalist. He is often given a fairly short deadline for completing articles (around 1–3 days). He became mildly depressed about six months ago and since then has had increasing difficulty meeting these deadlines. This has resulted in the following vicious cycles:

Thoughts:	*"I won't be able to write it properly."*
	"What if it's not good enough?"
	"I can't do this – I'm too anxious to even get started."
Feelings:	Anxious
	Low
Physical symptoms:	Tense, shaky
	Physically agitated – can't sit still
	Difficulty concentrating
Behaviour:	Puts off getting started until the last minute
	Eventually rushes through writing the article – standard may be lower

Keith's behavioural experiment planning chart

Alternative thought being tested: Just getting started by writing something about the subject, even if it is not very well written, might make me feel less anxious and help me write a better article

What am I going to do? (What, where, when...?)	For the next two weeks on alternate days, try the following two different strategies: 1. Continue current behaviour of putting off getting started until the last minute 2. Try a new strategy of doing 20 minutes of writing on the subject within an hour of receiving the brief. Pay no attention to 'quality' of writing at this stage – just write something about the subject Every day I will monitor how quickly I finish writing the brief, how anxious I feel during the day and how well written I think the finished article is.
What do I predict will happen?	I will spend 20 minutes writing complete rubbish and will feel even more frustrated afterwards.
What problems might arise with this plan?	Anxiety or panic may overcome me and I might not get started as quickly as planned.
How could these problems be overcome?	Turn computer on and sit at desk even if feeling anxious. Try to ignore anxious thoughts/feelings and just start writing anyway. Avoid distractions (e.g. don't turn TV on).
What happened when I tried the experiment?	*"On the days that I was trying the new approach I sometimes found it difficult to sit down and get started with my work but once I actually started writing it became much easier.* *On these days I managed to finish my article more quickly and felt less anxious. The article was often better as I had more time to write it.* *By the end of the 2 weeks, I had stopped putting off getting started, even on the days I was supposed to, because I could see it was making things worse."*

What have I learned from this experiment?
"Just getting started with the article, by writing something about the subject, helps me to finish it more quickly, and it is sometimes of a higher standard than when I am rushed. It is better to write something down, even if it is not perfect – this makes me feel less anxious and better able to get on with the task."

Case example 8.7: Finding time for enjoyable activities

Maria is 35-years old. She is married with 3 children and works part-time as an accountant. Maria is constantly trying to juggle the pressures of a busy job and her commitments to her family. Sometimes she feels anxious and low because she feels she is 'failing' to live up to her very high standards in all areas of her life. She drives herself hard and is very busy. She leaves little personal time to undertake enjoyable activities for herself alone.

Thoughts:	*"I have so much to do – there's no time for myself."*
	"I must constantly work hard."
	"Taking time for me is less important than all other responsibilities."
Feelings:	Anxious, tense
	Frustrated and easily irritated
	Occasionally low and tearful
Physical symptoms:	Agitated and tense
	Tired, mentally and physically
	Regular headaches
Behaviour:	Constantly 'on the go' around the home or catching up with work
	Has stopped doing many activities she used to enjoy (e.g. visiting friends, going to gym)
	Easily irritable and reacts by snapping at husband and children

Maria's behavioural experiment planning chart

Alternative thought being tested: Taking some time for myself will give me a much needed opportunity to relax and enjoy myself. Being happier and more relaxed and will help me get my other jobs done more effectively.

What am I going to do? (What, where, when...?)	Plan out enjoyable activities to carry out twice a week (e.g. taking long, relaxing bath, half-hour reading, meeting friend for coffee, going swimming).
What do I predict will happen?	Trying to fit in enjoyable activities will simply make me even busier and I will feel even more stressed and irritable. I will end up taking it out on my husband and children. I won't be able to enjoy the activities because I will be worrying about all the other things I have to do.
What problems might arise with this plan?	I may be too busy to get around to doing the activity. Other problems may get in the way, e.g. last-minute deadlines at work or a problem with the children.

How could these problems be overcome?	Decide in advance what I plan to do and when to do it. Plan some shorter sessions at convenient times (e.g. half-hour reading once children in bed) as well as longer times. Ask husband or sister to look after children. Be flexible – if last minute problem comes up, then re-schedule 'me-time' for next day (but make sure I don't keep putting it off).
What happened when I tried the experiment?	*"I was surprised how much I missed doing these kinds of activity and how much I enjoyed them. It was not easy to fit in everything but I did manage to fit in most of the planned activities.* *I also managed to fit in one evening at the cinema with my husband, which we haven't done for a long time.* *I felt happier afterwards and more relaxed and found that I was less irritable with my family. I still managed to get most of my other jobs done."*

What have I learned from this experiment?
"It is really important for me to have some enjoyable time – both alone and with my husband. It can get crowded out by all the other jobs, many of which are really not as important as they seem at the time. Taking 'me-time' helps me to relax and this improves my relationships with my family."

Reminders: Planning behavioural experiments

There are four key stages for planning behavioural experiments:
- Identify the problem: including relevant thoughts, negative predictions, feelings and existing behaviour)
- Plan changes to test out: a detailed, 'no-lose' plan which is realistic and acceptable to the patient and is relevant to the key negative beliefs being tested
- Try out the new behaviour and keep a written record of what happened
- Review and reflect on what the information means to the patient and how it can be used to improve life. This includes problem-solving to overcome any difficulties and planning relevant future experiments

Chapter 9

Overcoming practical problems: problem-solving approaches

- Problem-solving techniques help patients overcome practical or environmental problems

- Understanding and clarifying problems can make difficulties seem more manageable and increase a sense of control over life

- Learning a simple eight-step approach makes solving problems straightforward and can be used by patients to cope *themselves* with future difficulties

What is 'problem-solving'?

Problem-solving techniques offer a structured way to overcome real-life, practical problems and make changes in difficult environmental circumstances.

The benefit of problem-solving approaches does *not* depend entirely on solving the patient's problems. It can be therapeutic to simply identify what the problems actually are, making life seem more understandable and manageable. Using a problem-solving approach can give people a sense of hope, as well as an increased sense of control over their lives and problems. Problem-solving may also be beneficial by identifying helpful changes in behaviour. This can also have a positive effect on mood.

When to use a problem-solving approach

A problem-solving approach is useful when patients attribute many of their difficulties to the presence of practical problems and life stresses. Having to face a number of seemingly impossible problems can result in feelings of depression or anxiety. Patients may directly express concerns about life problems or it may become apparent through discussion of 'environmental factors' when working through different areas of the CBM (*Figure 9.1*).

Figure 9.1: Role of environmental factors in CBM

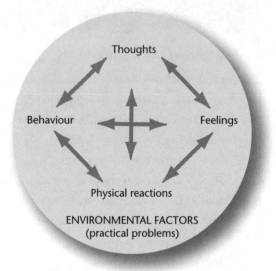

A problem-solving approach can be combined with making changes in other areas of the CBM, such as by altering unhelpful thoughts or behaviours that may be contributing to problems. For example, by improving depressed mood, people may feel less concerned or anxious about their ongoing life difficulties, or may gain the confidence to actively tackle and make changes in problem areas.

Reminders: What is problem-solving?

■ A problem-solving approach offers a structured way to understand and solve problems
■ The process of identifying and clarifying problems can be therapeutic in itself
■ Using problem-solving techniques can increase people's sense of control over their lives and problems
■ It can be helpful to combine a problem-solving approach with making changes in unhelpful thoughts or behaviour in relation to problems

Approaching problem-solving with patients

It is important to give a clear rationale and explanation of the problem-solving approach, as patients may have already unsuccessfully attempted to solve problems themselves or view them as completely impossible to change. This includes a brief overview of the approach and how it may help the patient:

"*Sometimes the problems in our lives can make us feel down or low, and may make life seem overwhelming or out of control. This approach can help to make sense of these problems and look for solutions to them. This might help to lift your mood and enable you to feel more in control of your life.*"

It is helpful to take a structured approach to problem-solving, which involves eight clearly defined steps (*Box 9.1*).

"*This is a very structured approach to solving problems: there are eight specific steps. It is important to carry out each of these steps in turn. Learning these steps means that you will be able to approach and solve any future problems in the same way.*"

Box 9.1: The eight steps of problem-solving

1. Make a list of problems
2. Choose a problem to address
3. Define the problem clearly
4. Generate solutions to problems
5. Choose a solution
6. Make an action plan
7. Carry out the plan
8. Review what happened

For effective problem-solving, it is particularly important to develop a collaborative relationship with patients, where they take an active role in the process. Potential solutions to problems should arise from patients rather than health professionals.

"*As these are your problems, you understand them better than anyone else. You are the most important person in this process, and it is vital that you do the 'work' by finding your own ideas and suggestions.*"

It is also useful to emphasize the need for 'homework'

> *"For this approach to actually improve things in your life, it is vital that you make real changes in your actions and behaviour. Without actually 'doing anything' about your problems, they are unlikely to change. Part of the problem-solving process is for you to try out some specific tasks or 'homework', which we will decide between us."*

Reminders: Approaching problem-solving with patients

- Begin by giving a clear explanation and rationale for a problem-solving approach
- Problem-solving involves a structured approach with eight specific steps
- A collaborative relationship is important, which encourages patients to take responsibility for solving their own problems
- 'Homework' translates discussions into real changes in a patient's life

The Eight Steps of Problem-Solving

Step 1: Make a list of problems

The first step involves identifying and making a written list of the patient's different problems.

> *"What problems are bothering you the most at the moment?"*

The aim is to get a broad overview of the important areas without going into too much detail.

> *"OK, you mentioned that you have some financial troubles and also not getting on too well with your husband. Are there any other important problems in your life at the moment?"*

The list should cover most key problem areas. It should include minor as well as major difficulties, as initially it is often easier to focus on less complex or difficult problems.

> *"You can also include smaller or less major problems on the list – sometimes it's helpful to solve the easier problems first."*

It is often useful to discover how these problems are affecting the patient. This helps to provide motivation to make changes. Remember to express empathy for the emotional distress associated with a patient's difficult life problems.

> *"How are these problems affecting your life? How do they make you feel?"*
>
> *"That sounds really difficult. It must be really distressing for you."*

Once the problem list is complete, it is useful to give the patient a brief summary of what they have told you.

> *"We have made a list of the practical problems that you are facing at the moment. You are having financial troubles with your mortgage, problems in your relationship with your partner and you have a difficult boss at work."*

"Tell me, have we got this right? Are these the most important issues that are facing you right now?"

Case example 9.1: Making a list of problems

Karen is a 27-year old nurse, who works part-time on a surgical ward in the local hospital. She has become mildly depressed over the past year. She is married and has two children aged 2 and 5. Karen's GP suggests that Karen might benefit from trying a problem-solving approach to understand and resolve some of the difficulties that she faces.

They begin by generating Karen's current problem list:

1. Unhappy at work – doesn't get on with ward manager
2. No time for herself – lack of enjoyable activities in her life
3. Health problems – recurrent back pain
4. Husband currently unemployed – financial difficulties

Reminders: Step 1 – Make a list of problems

- Make a written overview of all key problems faced by the patient
- Include more simple/minor problems as well as complex/major problems
- Identifying how these problems are affecting patients' lives, including how these difficulties make them feel emotionally, helps motivate patients to make changes
- Express empathy for difficulties and emotional distress described by patients
- Finish with a brief summary of the problem list

Step 2: Choose a problem to solve

The next step is for the patient to choose a problem to focus on first.

"Which of these problems would you be most interested in looking at in more depth?"

For problem-solving to be effective, the problem must:

- Involve an area which it is possible for the patient to change
- Be important to the patient

It is not necessary to start with the most complex or difficult problem.

"For the first attempt, it may be more helpful to choose a problem that is not too difficult, so that we are likely to be able to make some progress with it. This helps you to learn the technique and builds your confidence in using the approach. You could look at a more complex problem next time."

It is also important to focus on solving one problem at a time. However, some patients may feel that it is not 'enough'. Here, it may be helpful to discuss the advantages and disadvantages of changing one thing at a time versus trying to change everything at once. Use guided discovery to encourage the patient to come to their own conclusions.

Case example 9.2: Choosing a problem to solve

Let's return to the example of Karen, a 27-year old nurse, with mild depression. In the following dialogue, Karen and her GP discuss the pros and cons of changing one problem at a time:

GP Would you like to choose one of these problems to try to solve first?

Karen I'm not sure. I have so many problems, I'm not sure that changing one small thing will make any difference.

GP I see. Perhaps we could treat that as a *thought* to be tested out. It sounds like you are thinking that '*Changing one small thing won't make any difference to my problems.*'

Karen Yes, that's right.

GP What makes you think that is true? What is the evidence that is correct?

Karen I have so many problems at the moment. There doesn't seem much point in just looking at one small area.

GP OK – I will write that down. Anything else that makes you think that way?

Karen I feel so fed up, I'm not sure I can change anything anyway.

GP That's important to know. Any more reasons why you think that 'changing one thing won't make any difference'?

Karen Well, I think that some of the most important problems might not be possible to solve – I can't give my husband a job, for example.

GP I understand. I have written all these reasons down. Now, can you think of anything that might challenge or contradict the idea that 'changing one thing won't make any difference'? Is it possible that it could be helpful in any way?

Karen I suppose that it is still better to solve some problems, even if I can't solve them all.

GP Excellent. Anything else?

Karen I'm not sure.

GP How might it make you feel, to successfully solve some of your problems, even small ones?

Karen I would probably feel quite pleased with myself.

GP Yes, hopefully it would build up your confidence and boost your mood a bit. Do you think there might be any advantage in looking at one problem at a time? What might be the difficulties in trying to solve all your problems at once?

Karen It is probably impossible to solve everything at once. I probably wouldn't get very far and I might just give up and feel worse.

GP Great. Could you read through the evidence you have thought up, for and against the idea that 'changing one thing won't make any difference to my problems'. What do make of all this now?

Karen I can see that it does make sense to try to work on one thing at a time and that even improving one small thing might boost my spirits

GP Yes, that makes a lot of sense. Now, which problem would you like to look at first? Ideally, it should be something important to you and possible to change...?

Karen I am not very happy at work. Perhaps we should look at that.

GP OK, let's move onto the next step and talk about it in more depth....

Reminders: Step 2 – Choose a problem to solve

■ The patient chooses one problem area to focus on
■ The problem must be *important* to the patient as well as being *possible to change*
■ Avoid starting with the most complex or difficult problems

Step 3: Define the problem clearly

The problem must be clearly defined in precise and simple terms. It should be focused, specific and not too complex. Patients will often initially describe very broad, general problem areas. However, it often helpful to break these down into smaller, more manageable chunks:

General/broad problem: I am lonely and depressed

↓   ↓

Specific/focused/clear: I don't go out to any social events during the week

Encourage the patient to identify what specific 'chunks' would be most useful to look at first.

"You have described your problem in quite general terms. It is often easier to solve problems by breaking it down into smaller 'chunks' and working through one at a time."

"What are the most important parts of this problem? What exactly do you find difficult about...?"

For example, a patient may describe a problem of 'not having a girlfriend'. It might be helpful to break this down into specific areas, such as:

• Lack of social interaction (e.g. few friends or lack of regular social activities)

- Not meeting single women because of current lifestyle (e.g. working long hours)
- Lack of self-confidence (e.g. avoids talking to members of the opposite sex, anxiety about personal attributes or attractiveness)

For complex problems, it may also be necessary to break problems into *stages* that can be addressed sequentially to resolve the problem:

> *"It can be helpful to break problems into smaller 'steps' or 'stages, which can be looked at in turn. What might be the first step in solving your problem...?"*

Case example 9.3: Defining problems clearly

Let's return to the example of Karen, a 27-year old nurse, with mild depression. In the following dialogue, Karen and her GP discuss her work problems in order to define the problem clearly:

GP You mentioned your problems with work. Could you be a bit more specific about what exactly you find difficult?

Karen The main problem is that I don't have a good relationship with my ward manager. We are very short-staffed and she expects us to do extra shifts without much notice. But I just can't do that because I can't get childcare.

GP Is there anything else?

Karen Well, the manager can be quite bossy and critical. Several of my good friends have left the nursing team in the past year so I am not really enjoying working on that ward anymore.

GP I see. I made a note of the areas that you mentioned: you have a difficult relationship with your ward manager, the ward is short-staffed, you are expected to do extra shifts without notice, you find your manager bossy and critical and several of your friends have left the team in the past year. Is that right?

Karen Yes, that's it.

GP What would you like to achieve from solving this problem? What specific areas would you like to improve?

Karen I would like to enjoy my work again and have good relationships with my colleagues.

GP Great. I will make a note of that.

Reminders: Step 3 – Define the problem clearly

- Define the problem in precise and simple terms
- Break down broad or vague problems into specific 'chunks' or sequential stages to solve in turn
- Make a list of specific components of the problem
- Finish by asking the patient what they would like to achieve from solving the problem or what specific areas they would most like to change

Step 4: Generate solutions to problems

The next stage is to encourage the patient to think of a wide range of potential solutions to their problem. The patient must take an active role in leading the discussion and generating solutions.

First the patient must consider *what* they would like to achieve:

> *"What would need to change for you to feel better…?"*

Next, the patient must think creatively, or 'brainstorm' possible solutions for *how* to achieve this goal. The more solutions that are generated, the more likely a useful one will emerge. It is therefore useful to include a wide range of potential solutions, even if some ideas seem impractical or ridiculous. These 'wild' solutions could be adapted or modified to become workable, realistic possibilities.

> *"Can you think of any possible solutions to this problem?"*
>
> *"What other ideas can you think of? Try to think of as many possibilities as you can…"*
>
> *"What would your best friend/partner/boss/parent suggest? What advice would you give to a friend in the same situation?"*
>
> *"Can you think of any ridiculous or 'crazy' solutions as well as more sensible ones?"*

From Theory to Practice… Encouraging lateral thinking	It is possible to encourage lateral thinking using the 'brick technique' (Nezu & Nezu, 1989). Use the following example to encourage patients to think creatively and laterally about new ways to solve problems:
	Ask the patient to think up as many uses as possible for an item such as a house brick.
	Initially, the patient is likely to generate common, obvious suggestions such as building a house or a wall.
	Next, give the patient some other scenarios, to encourage them to think more laterally:
	• *"Could it have any other, more unusual uses?"*
	• *"Could it be used as a piece of furniture?"*
	• *"What if you became locked out of your car?"*
	• *"How might a child play with it?"*

Case example 9.4: Generating solutions to problems

Let's return to the example of Karen. Her GP encourages Karen to 'brainstorm' a wide range of possible solutions to her problem with work:

GP Can you think of any possible solutions to this problem?

continued

> **Karen** I'm not sure. I suppose I could try to work shifts where the ward manager is not on duty.
>
> **GP** That's a good start. Anything else?
>
> **Karen** I could look for a job on a different ward.
>
> **GP** Good. What advice would you give to someone else in the same situation?
>
> **Karen** I might suggest that they discuss their difficulties with childcare with their manager.
>
> **GP** OK, can you think of any really crazy or wild solutions to the problem? How else could you make your work more enjoyable?
>
> **Karen** Err... Well, I used to really enjoy chatting and laughing with my friends at work. I could throw a big party for all the ward staff to cheer them up!
>
> **GP** Great! Now, does that lead you to any other solutions which might help?
>
> **Karen** Actually, it might help me to get to know some of the new staff on the ward a bit better, maybe some kind of ward social event. We used to have them all the time.
>
> **GP** What exactly could you do to make this happen?
>
> **Karen** I could organize a ward night out. Or perhaps just invite a couple of the girls out for a drink after one of our shifts.

Reminders: Step 4 – Generate solutions to problems

- Identify what needs to change for the problem to improve
- Encourage the patient to generate a wide range of potential solutions to the problem
- 'Brainstorming' should include some impractical or ridiculous ideas as this helps the patient to think creatively and may lead to some useful, new possibilities
- Suggestions must arise from patients rather than health professionals

Step 5: Choose a solution

Once the patient has written a list of potential solutions, the next step is to consider each solution's advantages and disadvantages, in order to decide what action to take.

Box 9.2:
Assessing the value of potential solutions

> - How realistic or achievable is this solution likely to be?
> - How helpful is this solution is likely to be?
> - What are the pros and cons of each suggestion (e.g. time, effort, money, stress or other emotional distress)?
> - What positive or negative impact might this solution have on friends or family?

Again, most of these ideas should be generated by the patient. However, if the patient is overlooking a major advantage or disadvantage, then it can be helpful to bring it to their attention:

"Do you think it is important to take into account that....?"

After assessing each solution in turn, the patient must then choose the preferred solution(s) to try.

When reviewing the suitability of any solution, check it against the 'SMART' criteria (*Box 9.3*). This helps to ensure that the solution is realistic, workable and potentially useful for solving the patient's problem,

Box 9.3:
SMART criteria for goals and solutions

Is the solution:
Specific: clear definition of what the patient is going to do?
Measurable: easy to measure if the goal has been achieved or not?
Achievable: practical and realistic for the patient to carry out?
Relevant: useful and helpful to overcome the problem?
Timed: has a clearly defined timescale for carrying out the task?

If the patient's chosen solutions seem over-ambitious, it may be helpful to encourage them to break it down into smaller, more achievable 'chunks':

"This is a very interesting solution, but I am concerned it may be quite difficult for you to achieve all at once. Can you see any way to break it down into smaller pieces that might be easier to manage?"

Overly complex solutions may also indicate that the problem definition itself is too broad. In this case, return to Step 3 and break down the problem further into smaller sections or stages.

Case example 9.5: Assessing the advantages and disadvantages of solutions

Returning again to the previous case studies in this chapter, here is Karen's list of solutions:

Solution	Advantages	Disadvantages
Try to work shifts when ward manager is not on duty Look for another job on a different ward	Avoid being criticized or asked to work extra shifts New challenges Potentially better work environment	Difficult to manage – manager organizes rota May be worse than current job Have to get to know new environment/system Might be stressful

continued

Solution	Advantages	Disadvantages
Discuss childcare issues with ward manager	May stop her making unrealistic demands on my time Quick	Scary to talk to her – she could get angry Might not make any difference
Throw a big party for ward staff	Fun	Expensive Too much organization
Organize a ward night out	Get to know ward staff better	What if no one came? Difficult to coordinate with shifts of all staff
Invite a few people for a drink after work	Nice to get to know people Might make work more enjoyable if make friends	They might not want to come Would I be able to arrange childcare?

Choice of solution(s):
1. Discuss childcare issues with ward manager
2. Invite two people (Amanda and Jane) for coffee

Reminders: Step 5 – Choose a solution

- Ask patients to identify the advantages and disadvantages of each potential solution to the problem
- Next, patients should choose their preferred solution(s) to try
- Check that solutions fit the 'SMART' criteria and are realistic, achievable and useful

---

Step 6: Make an action plan

Once the solution has been chosen, the next stage is to draw up a written action plan and, being as specific as possible, write down exactly *what* the patient plans to do and *when* (*Box 9.4*).

Patients must understand what they need to do and feel comfortable and confident enough to try the solution out in practice.

Box 9.4: Steps for making an action plan

- What needs to be done?
- Where is it to be done?
- Who does it involve?
- How will it be done?
- When will it be done?
- What difficulties might arise and how will I cope with them?

"Are you clear about what you are going to do?"

"How confident are you that you will be able to carry this out?"

If they lack confidence in achieving the plan, the solution may need to be broken down into simpler steps.

"How could we change this plan to make it seem more manageable or realistic for you to achieve?"

It can also be helpful to consider what barriers might prevent patients from achieving a particular plan and to plan in advance how to overcome them:

"What might get in the way of being able to achieve this?"

"How could you overcome these difficulties?"

As with any other 'homework' task, it is important to establish any patient's commitment to carrying out the plan. Health professionals can encourage

---

Case example 9.6: Turning solutions into plans

Following on from Case example 9.5, here is Karen's action plan:

Solution	Action plan
Discuss childcare issues with ward manager	*Plan* • Ring ward manager in advance and ask her to arrange a time to discuss rota • Explain difficulties with child care and not able to do many 'ad hoc' shifts – request rota in advance to book child care arrangements *Possible difficulties* • Might feel nervous and get tongue-tied *How to overcome difficulties* • Plan what to say in advance and write it down
Invite two people (Amanda and Jane) for coffee	*Plan* • Look for a shift when both Amanda and Jane are on duty within next week • Suggest going for coffee after one morning shift in the next 2–3 weeks *Possible difficulties* • They might be busy or say no • Might not fit with my child care arrangements *How to overcome difficulties* • Be flexible about date, time and location • Be prepared to have coffee with one of them instead of both on the first occasion (could repeat another time if goes well)

patients by expressing interest in the outcome of the task, both beforehand and in a review consultation afterwards.

> *"Carrying out the plan is the most important step, because it can improve your problems. I will be really interested in hearing how you got on when I see you again in two weeks."*

It is helpful to create a *written* action plan, with a copy for both GP and patient to keep. Without this, the patient may forget what they are planning to do.

Reminder: Step 6 – Make an action plan

■ Draw up a written action plan of the specific steps to take to carry out the solution
■ Ensure the patient is clear about what they plan to do
■ Consider in advance what difficulties might arise with the plan and how to overcome them
■ Offering a follow-up appointment may help motivate the patient to carry out the task

---

Step 7: Carry out the plan

This is a self-explanatory step where the patient carries out the action plan.

Step 8: Review what happened

One of the most important stages of problem-solving is to reflect on what actually happened after trying out a solution. Remember to ask patients how they got on with any agreed solution or action plan. This gives a clear message that trying out the plan is important and necessary to solve problems.

> *"What happened when you tried...? I am so interested in hearing about it."*

Box 9.5:
Questions for reviewing the outcome of problem-solving action plans

- What did the patient do?
- Did it help to improve the problem? How?
- Were there any other positive outcomes?
- Were there any problems or difficulties with the approach?
- What can the patient learn from this?

It is important to encourage the patient by praising *any* success or positive outcome, however small. This helps boost the patient's confidence and self-belief in their ability to cope with difficulties.

Reviewing difficulties

If the patient found the action plan difficult to carry out or unhelpful in solving their problem, it is important to review these difficulties (*Box 9.6*).

Any difficulties encountered should be viewed as 'learning opportunities' rather than as 'failures'.

1. *Was the patient able to carry out the plan? How difficult was it to carry out?*
   If the patient found the action plan difficult or was unable to carry it out, ask:
   - Was the plan too ambitious or unrealistic?
   - What obstacles or barriers got in the way? How could these be overcome?
   - Did the patient lack motivation for the task? How could this be increased in future? What benefits might arise from solving this problem?
   - Was the problem less important than other issues in the patient's life that should be addressed first?

2. *How helpful was the plan in solving the problem?*
   If the plan was not helpful, review why this was the case:
   - Was the patient attempting to change something that was outside their control?
   - Was the solution not focussed on the most important part of the problem for the patient?
   - Is the problem still important to solve? If so, how could the patient change their approach to the problem?

Case example 9.7: Reviewing what happened

Karen returns to see her GP two weeks after trying out the problem-solving approach, to discuss what happened.

GP I am very interested to find out what happened with your plan to try and solve your problems at work...

Karen Well, I did try to carry out the plan that we agreed, but it wasn't very easy. I put it off until I knew I was coming back to see you!

GP It can sometimes be very difficult to make changes. Tell me, what happened?

Karen I was planning to do two things. One of them was quite easy. About 3 days after I saw you, I noticed that Jane and Amanda were both on duty with me. During our break, I suggested that we went for a coffee one day after work.

GP How did they respond to that?

Karen They both said they would really like to. They seemed pleased and we are due to go to a café next Wednesday. My husband has agreed to look after my children for a couple of hours, so it should be no problem.

continued

GP Great. How do you feel about this? Has it helped solve your problem with work at all?

Karen I'm pleased because I made the effort and it worked out. I hope that it might make work a bit more enjoyable if I know these people better.

GP Was it helpful in any other way at all?

Karen It will be nice to get my social life a bit more active, now that some of my friends have moved away from the area.

GP I am pleased that went well. What does this show you about your ability to solve your problems and improve life?

Karen It shows that I can make a difference, as long as I actually make the effort to do things.

GP I think that's absolutely right. You mentioned that the other part of the plan wasn't so easy. What happened?

Karen I was supposed to talk to my ward manager about my childcare problems but I didn't get around to it.

GP What stopped you from doing this?

Karen Well, she was away on holiday for the first week. Then, I didn't see her at all for quite a few days. By then, I had lost my nerve!

GP What do you mean by 'losing your nerve'? What were you concerned might happen?

Karen I was worried that she would get angry and shout at me.

GP I see. Is it still important to you to have this discussion with her? In what way would that actually help you?

Karen It is important because I want to make it clear that I just can't do all these extra shifts. I'm getting really stressed every time I see the rota and I want to sort it out.

GP So it is still something important to you to change?

Karen Yes it is.

GP How could you overcome this problem with 'losing your nerve'? What might help?

Karen I think it might help if I don't keep putting it off. She is back from holiday now so I should phone up and arrange to see her very soon.

GP Anything else?

Karen I could practice what I am going to say and write it down. I didn't do that last time.

GP Great. Is there any way to look at the situation that might make it seem less intimidating or scary?

Karen Well, I could imagine her naked!

GP That might work! How likely do you think it is that she will shout at you?

Karen Well, she might not actually shout at me at all.

GP Would it still be worth doing, even if she did get angry?

Karen Yes I think so, because this is a problem that is important to me to sort out. If she really is that unreasonable I would have to think more seriously about changing to a different ward.

GP I see. Let's make another action plan...

Figure 9.2: The problem-solving cycle

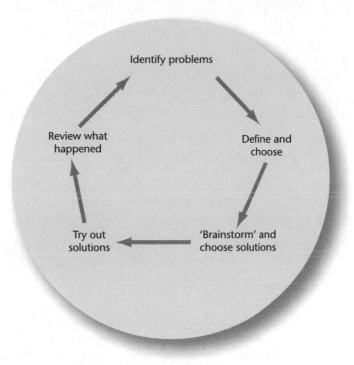

The problem-solving cycle

Problem-solving can be seen as an ongoing cycle of identifying problems, looking for solutions, and then reviewing the outcome of any changes made (*Figure 9.2*). This approach assumes that there may never be an 'absolute' solution to problems, but that life involves a continuous process of reflecting on difficulties and looking for solutions. This can make it less disheartening when one particular solution is unhelpful for a problem.

Reminders: Step 8 – Review what happened

- Reflecting on *what happened* after trying out solution to a problem is a key stage in the problem-solving process
- Reinforce and encourage *any* positive success to help motivate patients to persist when making changes
- Reflect on any difficulties that arose and try to identify ways to overcome these barriers to solving the problem

Chapter 10

Deeper levels of belief: core beliefs and rules

- Core beliefs and rules represent deep-seated beliefs, which are likely to have developed through early and significant life experiences

- They can be viewed as a system of 'roots' which underlie negative automatic thoughts and can be used to predict emotional distress in specific situations

- Changing these types of belief is a long and slow process, which may be difficult in primary care settings.

- Being aware of the presence of these beliefs in themselves and others can help GPs to understand and support patients more effectively

Different types of thought

CBT identifies three different levels of thought process: automatic thoughts, 'rules for living' and 'core beliefs' (*Figure 10.1*).

Automatic thoughts are the most 'superficial' level of thought. These are verbal messages or images that arise rapidly in response to events. They are the most accessible and easily identifiable type of thought, which 'pop' into people's minds throughout the day. A key CBT strategy is to teach patients to identify and find rational alternatives for negative automatic thoughts. This approach enables many patients to combat emotional disorders and improve mood.

A useful analogy is to compare the negative thoughts associated with severe emotional distress to the growth of weeds in a garden (Greenberger & Padesky, 1995b). Learning to identify and reframe any negative thoughts is like cutting down these weeds, allowing the flowers (helpful, alternative thoughts) to grow through. For many patients, this process is enough to learn to cope with their problems effectively.

However, negative automatic thoughts may reflect underlying, deeper levels of belief that people hold about themselves, other people and the world. It is sometimes necessary to remove weeds more permanently by digging down and taking them out by the root. By changing these underlying negative core beliefs and rules, people will reduce the number of negative automatic thoughts that are likely to arise in certain situations. Directly addressing such beliefs may also help with the process of changing unhelpful behaviour .

Figure 10.1:
Different types of
thought

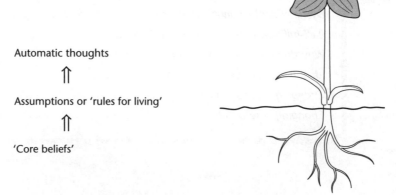

Automatic thoughts

⇑

Assumptions or 'rules for living'

⇑

'Core beliefs'

The deepest level thoughts are known as *core beliefs*. These types of beliefs include both positive and negative views of the self and the world. They are sometimes known as 'bottom line' beliefs as they may underpin more superficial negative automatic thoughts. Core beliefs involve absolutist statements that are usually expressed in black-and-white language such as:

"I'm stupid."	*"I'm clever."*
"I'm worthless."	*"I'm interesting."*
"I'm weak and vulnerable to illness."	*"I'm strong and healthy."*
"Others are not to be trusted."	*"Others are kind and supportive."*
"The world is a dangerous place."	*"Things always turn out well."*

Core beliefs are often acquired during childhood and early life; they represent people's enduring understanding of themselves and their world. This understanding is necessary in order to help people make sense of their experiences and to react appropriately to events.

'Rules for living' are a set of rules that guide people's expectations of themselves and others. They can often be expressed as 'should' statements or as conditional, 'if...then...' statements.

"I should never make any mistakes."

"If I feel any physical symptoms then it means there is something seriously wrong."

"If I don't please others at all times then they will reject me."

"If people don't agree with me then it means that they don't respect me."

"I should always be in control."

'Rules for living' often develop in order to help people live with 'tyrannical', absolutist, negative core beliefs. There are often two paired beliefs for each rule, which illustrate a person's beliefs about how they 'should' behave, as well as outlining the consequences or meaning if the rule is broken. For example, a person with the negative core belief *'I'm a failure'* may develop the following pair of rules:

"If I do everything perfectly then it means that I am OK."

"If I make a mistake it means I am a total failure."

Whilst automatic thoughts are often stated directly in people's minds, rules may be less obvious. However, they can often be inferred from people's actions or reactions to particular situations. People are often not consciously aware of the rules themselves, but are aware of the emotional discomfort that arises from transgressing them. If people's rules are, or are *at risk* of being broken, they are likely to develop a negative emotional response associated with a host of negative automatic thoughts. This explains an apparent 'over-reaction' that a person may experience when faced by a seemingly minor event. For example, if someone holds perfectionist beliefs about potential failure, they are likely to feel extremely anxious in situations where this rule is threatened, such as taking an exam or any situation where they perceive there is a significant possibility of making a mistake. They may react by *avoiding* such situations or alternatively by working excessively hard to try to ensure continual 'success'.

Case example 10.1: The development of core beliefs and rules for living

Anna was a quiet child. She was slightly overweight and wore glasses. She was often teased by the other children at school, who called her 'Specky-four-eyes'. Anna worked hard at school and often achieved good grades. However, whenever she was praised by teachers, her classmates would tease her, saying she was a 'boring, stuck-up, teacher's pet'.

As a consequence, Anna developed the core belief: "*I am unacceptable to others.*"

As Anna became older, she remained shy but developed a number of friendships. In response to these new experiences, she developed the following 'rules for living':

"*If someone doesn't like me then it means that I'm unacceptable.*"

"*If everyone likes me then it means that I am OK.*"

These rules make it easier for Anna to cope with her negative core belief. So long as everyone likes her then she is able to believe that her core belief is not true. However, if this rule is threatened or broken then she returns to believing her negative, 'bottom line' belief of being unacceptable.

Because of her beliefs, Anna is vulnerable to feeling especially low or upset whenever she suspects that someone might not like her. To prevent this, she often avoids threatening situations, such as meeting new people. She feels anxious and uncomfortable in social situations and experiences many negative, automatic thoughts about her own performance and the reactions of others such as:

"*Did I say something stupid?*"

"*I don't have anything interesting to say to anyone.*"

"*This person thinks I am too quiet and boring.*"

"*I should just go home – there is no point being here.*"

The first stage of improving Anna's self-esteem is to learn to identify and evaluate these negative automatic thoughts. Later, however, Anna may also benefit from learning methods of gradually changing the rules and core beliefs that underlie her difficulties.

Reminders: Different levels of thought

- Automatic thoughts are the most accessible and superficial level of thought – verbal messages or images that pop into people's minds in response to events
- Core beliefs are the deepest level of thought, which are usually absolutist statements expressed in black-and-white language
- Rules for living comprise a set of implicit rules that guide people's expectations of themselves and others. They are usually expressed as 'should' or conditional, 'if...then...' statements

Where do rules and core beliefs come from?

Rules and core beliefs usually arise from past experience. Many are also reinforced by cultural or gender stereotypes (e.g. perfectionism is associated with achievement). Many core beliefs develop during childhood and early life. The particular environment in which a child develops plays a strong role in shaping which beliefs are developed. For example, depending on their early experiences, a child may acquire beliefs such as "*Dogs will bite*" or "*Dogs are friendly.*"

The simplistic, absolutist quality of core beliefs reflects this kind of early, childhood learning. Although these beliefs are not necessarily *absolutely* true, young children do not have the mental capacity to think in flexible ways and tend to view them as absolute fact. Children may also view subjective statements about themselves or others (e.g. "*I am bad*"), as being just as certain or 'true' as other, more factually-based beliefs (e.g. "*Fire is dangerous*").

In later life, we learn to view most of these beliefs more flexibly. For example, we may learn to approach dogs that are wagging their tails and avoid those that are growling or appear aggressive. However, some of the old, absolute beliefs may remain. This is particularly likely if they developed from particularly traumatic experiences or if the beliefs are reinforced by ongoing life experiences.

Understanding how particular core beliefs and rules operate in individual patients can help to predict reactions or explain recurring themes of emotional distress in response to particular types of situation.

The development of these beliefs is illustrated in *Figure 10.2*.

Reminders: Where do core beliefs and rules come from?

■ Rules and core beliefs usually arise from past experience and may be reinforced by cultural or gender stereotypes
■ Young children develop simplistic beliefs that make sense of their experiences and often view these beliefs as *absolute fact*
■ The simplistic, absolutist quality of core beliefs reflects their development in early life
■ Rules for living usually develop in order to help the individual live with 'tyrannical' absolutist core beliefs

---

Dysfunctional or unhelpful rules and core beliefs

Everyone holds a set of rules and core beliefs, which help us to understand and live in the world by allowing us to generalize from our experiences. This ability enables us to apply our knowledge in different situations. For example, once we have learned to drive in one particular car, we are able to generalize this knowledge, so that we can also drive a new, unfamiliar car with little difficulty. However, if we get in a car which is markedly *different*,

Figure 10.2:
Development of
core beliefs and
rules

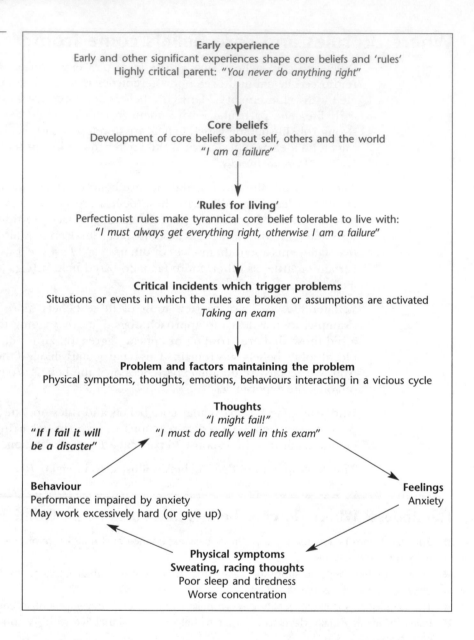

Early experience
Early and other significant experiences shape core beliefs and 'rules'
Highly critical parent: *"You never do anything right"*

Core beliefs
Development of core beliefs about self, others and the world
"I am a failure"

'Rules for living'
Perfectionist rules make tyrannical core belief tolerable to live with:
"I must always get everything right, otherwise I am a failure"

Critical incidents which trigger problems
Situations or events in which the rules are broken or assumptions are activated
Taking an exam

Problem and factors maintaining the problem
Physical symptoms, thoughts, emotions, behaviours interacting in a vicious cycle

Thoughts
"I might fail!"
"I must do really well in this exam"

**"If I fail it will
be a disaster"**

Behaviour
Performance impaired by anxiety
May work excessively hard (or give up)

Feelings
Anxiety

Physical symptoms
Sweating, racing thoughts
Poor sleep and tiredness
Worse concentration

such as 'left-hand drive', we may make mistakes because our *old* knowledge of driving is not fully applicable within the new environment. The more ingrained the knowledge, the more difficult it is to adjust to new circumstances.

Core beliefs and rules are often both *functional* and *adaptive* when they first develop. For example, a child who grows up in a violent, abusive or unpredictable environment may believe that, *"Bad things that happen are my fault"* and *"If I don't do anything wrong then bad things may not happen."* These beliefs may help the child to cope in that environment, rather than risking further abuse or rejection from his parents. Blaming themselves for negative events around them may also give children a sense of control which may be preferable to feeling helpless and powerless. There may also be an increased sense of security for children in believing that adults are 'good', even if this entails viewing themselves as 'bad'.

Core beliefs and rules are viewed as *dysfunctional* or *unhelpful* if they exert a negative or unhelpful effect on the person's life. On the whole, the more extreme and autocratic the rule, the less helpful it is likely to be. Dysfunctional beliefs arise when beliefs or rules are not adjusted or revised in the face of new evidence from later experience. In this way, early beliefs may persist despite being no longer fully applicable to people's ongoing environment and circumstances. Problems arise when people continue to view these beliefs as 100% accurate rather than simply beliefs generated during childhood. Such beliefs should be viewed as 'out of date' or 'unhelpful' rather than 'wrong'.

The level of belief in particular rules or core beliefs may vary. For many people, these types of core belief and rule may be activated only at certain times, such as periods of stress, low mood or in the presence of strong psychosocial pressures. In some enduring disorders, such as personality disorders, it is likely that powerful, negative core beliefs and rules are active for much of the time.

Reminders: Unhelpful or dysfunctional core beliefs and rules

- Rules and core beliefs help people to make sense of the world, enabling them to generalize from experience and apply their knowledge in different situations
- When core beliefs and rules develop during childhood, they are often designed to help the child cope in the particular environment in which they are growing up
- Core beliefs and rules become *dysfunctional* when they are no longer applicable to people's ongoing life circumstances and exert a negative or unhelpful impact on people's lives

---

'Self-fulfilment' of rules and core beliefs

Holding a particular rule or core belief is often 'self-fulfilling'. People often behave '*as if*' these beliefs are absolute fact. This usually reinforces the negative belief. For example, a woman who holds the rule, "*I must always put others ahead of me so they don't see what a bad person I am,*" is likely to behave in ways that that allow other people to dominate or treat her as a 'doormat'. This is likely to reinforce her belief that others think she is a bad person.

This kind of behaviour also prevents people from testing out the possibility that the negative belief may not actually be true. For example, the belief that "*If I spend time with others they will discover how boring I am and reject me,*" may lead to avoidance of contact or interaction with other people. While this may seem like the 'safest' option, it also means that the person is never able to discover that the rule is not completely accurate.

The presence of deeply held negative beliefs influences how people perceive the world. For example, a belief that "*I am inferior to others*" is usually based on numerous examples from someone's life, such as times that they have been ignored or badly treated by others. Someone holding this type of belief is likely to be highly sensitive and quick to notice experiences that confirm this perceived inferiority. Each negative experience is viewed as confirmation that their belief is true.

People holding negative beliefs are also likely to discount or ignore numerous examples of contradictory information. Core beliefs and rules usually have an absolute, black-and-white content, which rarely fits the reality of the world. It is almost impossible to be a *total* failure or *completely* worthless. These beliefs are maintained by *distorting* the facts to fit the belief and by *ignoring* contradictory information. For example, a person holding the core belief that "*I am unlikeable,*" is unlikely to suddenly change this negative view, even after meeting someone who behaves in a very positive or friendly way. Instead, they often discount this contradictory experience, by saying "*They probably didn't mean it. Maybe he wanted something from me or else just felt sorry for me.*" Alternatively, they may simply ignore, fail to notice or quickly forget his friendly behaviour. Padesky (1993) viewed this type of belief as an example of *self-prejudice*.

Case example 10.2: Viewing unhelpful beliefs as 'self-prejudice'

In the following dialogue, Valerie and her GP discuss her negative self-beliefs:

GP You mentioned that you are sometimes very critical of yourself, much more than with other people. If even small things go wrong, you often view yourself as a 'complete failure'.

Valerie Yes, that's right. I am very hard on myself.

GP One way to look at this is to see it as a form of 'prejudice'. Imagine for a moment, a very sexist man who believes that 'All women drivers are terrible.' One day he is walking down the street and he sees a woman driver having difficulty parking her car. She finishes by crashing into the car ahead. What would be his likely reaction?

Valerie He would probably say, "That's typical of a woman driver. They can't park. They shouldn't be on the road!"

GP Yes, that's right. It would confirm his idea that all women are bad drivers. The next day, this same sexist man, is walking down the road, when a woman does a perfect reverse park into a space in front of him. What is his likely reaction this time?

Valerie He'd probably say, "Well, she was lucky that time."

GP Yes, he might well say that. What other reaction might he have? Think about how many women there must be driving past him every day without crashing.

Valerie He might not even notice that she parked well.

GP Exactly right. So he might discount it by saying she was lucky or he might ignore it altogether. How could you tie in this idea with your own negative, self-critical thoughts?

Valerie I can see that I am very quick to notice everything that goes wrong, but I don't always register when things go well or I might discount the good things that I do.

GP How could you get around this problem? What could you do to make things a little more balanced and fair to yourself?

Valerie I could try to notice and remember the things that I do well.

GP That sounds like a really good idea. How can you make sure that you do remember these things?

Valerie I suppose I could write them down in a diary.

GP I would be really interested to see what you find out if you try doing that for a while.

Reminders: Self-fulfilment of rules and core beliefs

- By behaving 'as if' negative rules and core beliefs are absolute fact, they often become reinforced in reality
- By behaving in this way, people are unable to discover that the negative belief may not be completely accurate
- When people hold deep-rooted negative beliefs they become highly sensitive to information which confirms these beliefs but may discount or ignore any contradictory information
- Such beliefs can be understood as examples of self-prejudice

Why do GPs need to know about core beliefs and rules?

In CBT, it is usually more helpful to begin by working with the more accessible automatic thoughts, which are easier to change using thought records and verbal reattribution techniques. Only later, if negative thoughts recur persistently, is it appropriate to begin to work with the more complex and deeply held core beliefs and rules.

When activated, deeper level beliefs can be extremely powerful and are much more difficult to challenge and reframe than automatic thoughts. The process may be time consuming and require extensive, in-depth emotional work, which is often more appropriately carried out during a prolonged course of CBT. It may not be appropriate to work on these kinds of deep-seated belief within the time-limited setting of a GP consultation.

It is important for GPs and other health professionals to understand how deeper level beliefs develop and operate, because:

- Understanding the role of core beliefs and rules gives GPs a greater depth of understanding and insight into an individual patient's reactions and behaviour
- Identifying the presence of particular rules and core beliefs can help to predict people's future reactions to specific events. Altering these rules may reduce the risk of future relapse when faced by challenging life circumstances.
- The presence of deep-rooted beliefs may explain why methods of re-framing negative thoughts have proved unhelpful in certain patients.
- Identifying the presence of powerful core beliefs and rules can help GPs to make decisions about referrals for further CBT.
- Identifying the GP's own personal rules may be valuable for understanding our own negative emotional reactions to work-related and personal difficulties.

Maintaining emotional safety for patients

Deeply held, negative core beliefs can be extremely powerful and, when activated, can stimulate a great deal of unpleasant emotion. It is important for health professionals to be sensitive to any cues that suggest a patient is experiencing emotional discomfort and express empathy for their distress. It is also important to avoid arguing with patients about the 'best' or 'right' beliefs to hold. Remember that the patient is likely to have held these kinds of belief for many years. Such beliefs may be unhelpful but they may also seem familiar and 'safe'. It can be very threatening to face an entirely new way to view the world.

Reminders: Why do GPs need to know about core beliefs?

- Deeper level thoughts and beliefs are more difficult to challenge and reframe than automatic thoughts
- Their presence may explain why changing automatic negative thoughts are sometimes unhelpful in alleviating a patient's emotional distress
- Understanding the role of specific core beliefs and rules in individual patients may help to predict future behaviour/reactions to specific events
- Identifying a GP's own personal rules may also be valuable

Identifying core beliefs and rules

Core beliefs and rules may become apparent from particular, recurring themes that arise and result in emotional distress. For example, a person may experience anxiety in relation to any risk of potential 'failure'.

Another way to identify rules and core beliefs is to ask patients directly about the impact of their early life experiences:

"What conclusions did you draw about yourself or others, based on your early experiences in life?"

"How might this influence the problems you are experiencing right now?"

Core beliefs and rules can also be identified using the *downward arrow technique*. Instead of accepting thoughts at face value, this involves peeling away the layers of thoughts, beliefs and meaning to find out what lies beneath the patient's automatic negative thoughts and fears. This is equivalent to 'digging up' the roots of a weed, instead of just trimming the leaves growing above ground. The aim is to gently question the basis for any negative thoughts (*"If that really did happen, what would it mean to you...?"*)

Box 10.1:
Questions for
the 'downward
arrow'
technique

- *"If that thought were true, what would it mean to you?"*
- *"What's so bad about that?"*
- *"What does this situation say about you? What's the worst part about that?"*

Case example 10.3: Downward arrow technique

Dr T has been a GP for three years. He recently completed a diploma in diabetes management. He has been asked to run a workshop for a group of local GP colleagues on diabetes. The prospect of this presentation fills Dr T with dread. He has always hated giving talks to colleagues. On this occasion, he feels anxious and afraid and experiences the following negative automatic thoughts:

"What right do I have to speak to all these experienced GPs? Maybe I don't know enough about the subject."
"What if they don't agree with me or ask me questions that I can't answer?"
"I might look really foolish."
"What if I get so nervous I can't speak properly and can't get my point across?"

Dr T decides to discuss his fears about making the presentation with a mentor and they agree that it might be helpful to identify any underlying 'rules' which might explain his reaction.

Dr T When I think about giving the presentation, I get very anxious. I start thinking, 'What right do I have to speak to all these experienced GPs?' and 'What if they ask me something that I don't know the answer to?'
Mentor If that really did happen, if they asked you something that you didn't know the answer to, what would that mean about you?
Dr T Well, I might just stand there, looking really foolish...
Mentor And if that happened? What would that mean?

continued

> **Dr T** It would show that I wasn't fully in control. I wasn't prepared enough.
> **Mentor** What would be the worst bit about that?
> **Dr T** It would show that I don't really know what I'm talking about. I'm not as much of an expert as they might expect.
> **Mentor** And if that were true...?
> **Dr T** I'd be shown up as being incompetent.
> **Mentor** I see. Has this kind of belief come up with you before? Is there some kind of rule that you hold about this?
> **Dr T** I guess that I sometimes feel a bit of a fake. I get really anxious if I think people might 'find me out'
> **Mentor** And they might find out that...?
> **Dr T** That I don't really know what I'm doing, that I'm incompetent.
> **Mentor** Let's try and work out the exact wording of this rule. For most people it is an 'if...then...' or a 'should...' statement.
> **Dr T** I think it's that *'If I don't always appear completely in control, then people will realize I'm incompetent'*

Reminders: Identifying core beliefs and rules

- Core beliefs and rules may become apparent from particular, recurring themes that result in patients' emotional distress
- They can also be identified by asking directly about the impact of patients' early life experiences on their view of themselves as an adult
- The downward arrow technique involves 'digging' down to find out what lies beneath the patient's automatic negative thoughts and fears

From Theory to Practice...	What particular situations do you associate with your own 'heartsink' responses? Think of a recent example. What automatic thoughts arose during that situation?
	Now try the 'downward arrow' technique to try to identify what unhelpful rules might underlie your response.
	Ask yourself: *'If these negative thoughts are really true, what does that mean about me...?'*

Changing unhelpful rules

Simply identifying and clarifying the unspoken rules that guide people's behaviour can help some patients to begin to undermine and change their unhelpful rules. The first step is therefore to identify the precise wording of the rule using a method such as the downward arrow technique.

Some rules are examples of 'unhelpful thinking styles'. For example, perfectionist beliefs are usually examples of black-and-white thinking and could be reframed as a 'shades of grey' approach. Similarly, 'should' statements can are more helpfully changed to 'would prefer…' statements. It is more helpful to view rules as a guide to preference, rather than an absolute, unrealistic statement about how the world *must* be.

The process of working with rules is similar to the process of evaluating and reframing thoughts, discussed in Chapter 7. The aim is to identify the belief and then look for a wide range of evidence both for and against it being accurate or realistic. Remember that rules may have been held for some time and the collection of evidence should reflect this. It is also helpful to include a cost/benefit analysis of holding the rule. The final step is to identify an alternative, more balanced rule. This should be a more realistic perspective which retains the advantages of the old rule, while avoiding some of the disadvantages.

Include an assessment of the level of belief in each particular rule (*"How much do you believe this rule, from 0 to 100?"*) Remember that the aim is not to eliminate the rule entirely, but to reduce the level of belief in it, so that it exerts a less powerful effect over people's lives.

Box 10.2:
Evaluating rules and generating helpful alternatives

Evidence 'for' the old rule	Evidence 'against' the rule
What is the evidence that this rule is accurate or correct? What experiences in your life have proved it to you? What are the advantages of this rule? Are there any ways that it helps you to achieve your goals? What past experiences might have contributed to the development of this rule?	What is the evidence *against* this rule? Have you had any experiences which contradict it or which show that it is inaccurate or untrue? Is the rule unfair or unrealistic in any way? What are the disadvantages of this rule? How does it cause problems for you?

Generating a balanced alternative rule:

What could be a more helpful and realistic alternative to this rule? How could you maintain the advantages of the rule whilst minimizing the disadvantages?

Case example 10.4: Evaluating rules and generating helpful alternatives

Dr O is a GP who prides herself on having good relationships with her patients. She feels particularly stressed and anxious after seeing Nigel, a 45-year old man with chronic fatigue syndrome. He can be demanding and critical of his care from the practice staff.

continued

He presents to the surgery one day, and insists upon a neurology referral, which Dr O is unwilling to comply with. The result is a somewhat confrontational consultation, and Nigel leaves the surgery angrily. Dr O feels anxious and low. She identifies the following negative automatic thoughts:

"I didn't manage the situation well enough."

"I should have been able to deal it better. I didn't communicate with him well enough."

"I made a complete mess of this."

Dr O realizes that she often feels anxious and low if she feels that she has made a mistake or not 'performed' well enough. To identify her underlying rules, Dr O asks herself:

- *"If these thoughts were true, what would it mean about me?"*
- *"What does this situation say about me? What's the worst part about that?"*

Using the downward arrow technique, Dr O identifies the following rule: *'I must do everything perfectly; otherwise it means that I'm a complete failure'.*

Dr O fills out the following chart, to evaluate this rule and come up with a more helpful, alternative way to view the situation:

Old rule:
I must do everything perfectly; otherwise it means that I'm a complete failure

Evidence *for* this belief	Evidence *against* this belief
"At school and medical school, it was very important to do well." *"In childhood, my mother used to get upset if I failed an exam or didn't achieve very high marks"* *"There could be a very serious implication from making a mistake as a doctor."* *"Other people may think less of me if I make mistakes or appear imperfect."* *"Patient expectations are very high and litigation may follow if I make a mistake."* *"It feels great when I do well."* *"This rule helps me to succeed in life – it drives me on to work hard and do well."*	*"Absolute perfection is impossible to achieve."* *"Many successful people fail in some areas of their lives."* *"Many successful doctors fail the odd exam in medical school."* *"It's unrealistic to blanket all mistakes together – there are many different degrees."* *"I have made plenty of minor mistakes throughout my life and most of them did not lead to major disaster."* *"The most important thing is to learn from mistakes rather than be self-critical and label myself as a total failure."* *"I would never be this harsh on anyone else."* *"Everyone makes mistakes sometimes – it is normal and human."*

continued

"My mother got upset when I didn't do well because she loved me and thought I had great potential, not because she thought I was a failure."

New rule:
It is important to work hard at being 'good enough,' but making small mistakes or not being completely perfect is normal and human.

From Theory to Practice... Think back to your own personal rule that you identified during the previous 'From Theory to Practice' reflective exercise (p. 174).

Work through the process of gathering evidence for and against the rule. Remember to include a cost–benefit analysis of the rule.

What could be a more helpful rule? How could you begin to implement this rule in your daily life?

What would you do differently if you believed this new, alternative rule completely? Can you behave 'as if' the new rule is true?

Using behavioural experiments to overcome unhelpful rules

One of the most powerful ways of altering unhelpful rules is to use behavioural experiments. This creates a deeper level of belief than simply using verbal reattribution techniques.

Box 10.3: Examples of useful behavioural experiments

Unhelpful rule	Behaviour associated with rule	New rule to test	Ideas for experiments
I must always be in control.	Avoid situations where feel out of control. Behave in a dominant or aggressive manner with others to try to keep control of situations.	It is impossible to be in control of everyone and everything at all times. It is often helpful to allow other people to take responsibility for things too.	Try participating in situations without trying to take control. Notice what happens to stress levels and reactions from others.
If I don't please others at all times then they will reject me.	Put others first at all times and ignore own needs.	I deserve to spend some time meeting my own needs as well as those of other people.	Try putting aside some time in the week for enjoyable activities. Learn to say 'no' when necessary. Observe impact on self and others.

Box 10.3: *continued*

Unhelpful rule	Behaviour associated with rule	New rule to test	Ideas for experiments
If I don't try then I can't fail.	Avoid challenges and opportunities. Make little effort to achieve goals.	Trying new things is the only way to make achievements. It's not a disaster if things don't go as I wish, but avoiding things means I may miss out on some great opportunities.	Try out learning a new skill or aiming towards a new, positive goal.
If I avoid others then they will never find out how awful I am really	Avoid contact with other people. Withdrawn and isolated.	Other people may like me if I give them the opportunity to get to know me better.	Gradually test out having more contact with other people. Try talking and interacting more with others and see what happens.

Once the overall aim of the experiment has been identified, it is helpful to plan out a series of smaller steps to test out in practice. Rules can be tested with a range of different experiments.

Case example 10.5: Testing out unhelpful rules with behavioural experiments

Old rule: I must do everything perfectly; otherwise it means that I'm a complete failure

The following behavioural experiments show two different ways to test out and reframe this unhelpful rule.

First new rule to test: Making a small mistake doesn't cancel out all my good achievements

What could I do to test if this rule is really true? (What, where, when…?)	Make a list of my achievements. Then make a list of things that I have not done perfectly or mistakes I have made and what happened afterwards. I could then check to see if the mistakes completely outweigh the achievements and if they resulted in major disaster for me.

continued

What do I predict will happen?	I will realize how important it is to avoid mistakes, as I will remember all the terrible things that happened when I made mistakes.
What problems might arise with this plan?	It might make me feel anxious and stressed to think about any mistakes I have ever made.
How could these problems be overcome?	Make sure I spend plenty of time listing achievements before thinking of mistakes.
What happened when I tried the experiment?	*"I have made plenty of mistakes in my life, but most of them caused no major problems. Some things, which seemed to be problems at the time, actually worked out better in the end."*

What have I learned from this experiment? What is the new, more helpful rule?

"It really isn't always a disaster if things don't go completely perfectly. This happens often in life, and usually the problems are overcome in the end."

Second new rule to test: I will still be 'good enough' if I work less hard and keep time for enjoyable activities

What could I do to test if this rule is really true? (What, where, when...?)	Stop working at weekends for three weeks. Plan enjoyable activities instead. Then check with a work colleague about my work performance.
What do I predict will happen?	I won't achieve enough and colleagues will complain about me.
What problems might arise with this plan?	If an important project arises with a deadline that I have to meet urgently.
How could these problems be overcome?	Try to prioritize my work and get the most important jobs done during the week. As a last resort, work on Sunday afternoon if urgent deadline for Monday.
What happened when I tried the experiment?	*"I didn't need to work at the weekend. I got most of my work done during the week. My work colleagues didn't notice any change in my performance but noticed I seemed more relaxed and happy."*

What have I learned from this experiment? What is the new, more helpful rule?

"I can still be good at my job even if I don't spend all my weekends working. I am also a lot happier if I make time in my life for enjoyable activities as well."

Reminders: Changing unhelpful rules

■ Identifying and clarifying the unspoken rules that guide people's behaviour can help some patients to begin to undermine and change any unhelpful rules
■ Unhelpful rules can be evaluated by looking for evidence both for and against them being accurate or true
■ Behavioural experiments are one of the most powerful ways to generate evidence to disprove the old rule and test out alternative, more helpful rules

Changing core beliefs

As described above, core beliefs are usually absolutist, black-and-white beliefs about the self, others or the world. Changing core beliefs is a very long process, as they were usually learned in early life and have been reaffirmed by gathering evidence over a very long period of time. It involves gathering data to counteract a negative core belief, by noting down any experiences that support a more positive belief about the self or others. It may take weeks, months or even years to gather enough data.

The new core belief should be a more realistic and fair view of the world, rather than an equally unrealistic positive belief. For example, the negative core belief *"I'm worthless"* might be more helpfully reframed as *"I am good enough"* or *"I have plenty of worth as a person"*.

To slowly shift a core belief, an individual patient needs to keep track of as much evidence as possible that contradicts the old belief and supports the new one. This should include evidence from the past, as well as continuing to monitor for positive events, perhaps using a journal to record the data.

Box 10.4:
Questions for developing new core beliefs

- What things in your past contradict this belief?
- Are you ignoring or discounting any positive events which might support a more positive view of things?
- Can you keep an eye out for *any* situations that might support a more positive view?

Reminders: Changing core beliefs

■ Changing core beliefs is a long process, which involves gathering data to counteract the negative belief
■ The patient should identify and record past and present experiences that support a more positive belief about the self or others.
■ The new core belief should be a fairer and more realistic view of the world

Chapter 11

Anxiety and panic disorder

- Panic is associated with the catastrophic misinterpretation of the meaning of harmless physical symptoms

- Reducing panic involves giving patients credible, alternative explanations for their symptoms

- The CBM is a useful tool for explaining the nature of anxiety and fear

- The CBM can be used to increase patients' awareness of the role of cognitive and behavioural factors in anxiety and panic

- The CBM is useful for helping patients to learn to appraise potentially dangerous situations more realistically without getting into the vicious cycles of panic attacks

Understanding Anxiety

General principles of anxiety disorders

What is anxiety?

Anxiety is an unpleasant emotional state associated with *fear* and *unwanted distressing physical symptoms*. It is a normal and appropriate response to stress but becomes pathological when the reaction is extreme and disproportionate to the severity of the stress.

In anxiety states, the fear relates to some kind of future *danger*. This may be an immediate risk, such as during panic attacks, when people may fear having a heart attack and dying. It could also reflect a longer-term risk, such as in health anxiety, where people fear the future consequences of a possible severe illness. The focus of the danger can also be broken into *internal* and *external* factors. Internal dangers can be physical, such as having a stroke or heart attack or mental, such as losing control or going 'crazy'. External dangers include psychosocial risks such as the loss of a job or being perceived negatively by others.

The CBM is useful in anxiety disorders, where people are acutely aware of physical and emotional feelings of anxiety but may be less aware of the important role of thoughts, behaviour and environmental factors.

Characteristic unhelpful thinking styles in anxiety

Anxious people often have *catastrophic thoughts* where they overestimate the risk or likelihood that something bad will happen as well as focusing on the worst possible outcome of events. People also tend to underestimate their ability to cope if the feared event did take place.

From Theory to Practice...	To illustrate how anxious people tend to overestimate the risk and severity of danger, you could use an example, such as:

Imagine you are alone in the house late at night. Everything is quiet and dark. As you get into bed you hear a clatter downstairs. You immediately fear it is a burglar. Your heart races, your palms feel sweaty and you feel scared. Creeping downstairs you discover that it is just your cat – it has knocked over the bin! Your fear quickly dies away.

This is an example of overestimating the danger. Thoughts of danger can cause strong feelings of anxiety *even if* this danger is not real.

In anxiety or panic attacks, people often misinterpret an event as being more dangerous than it really is. This could involve misinterpreting the meaning of harmless physical symptoms (*"My heart is racing – I must be having a heart attack!"*) or perhaps seeing the disapproval of others as another type of catastrophe (*"They will think I am crazy and lose all respect for me"*).

Reminders: General principles of anxiety disorders

■ Anxiety is characterized by *fear* of a future *danger*
■ The danger might be a physical risk such as having a stroke or heart attack or a psychological risk such as a fear of going 'crazy'
■ Anxiety is associated with *catastrophic* thinking styles, where people overestimate the likelihood that a particular danger might occur and imagine the most disastrous outcome
■ Anxious patients often underestimate their own ability to cope with potential dangers

Understanding panic disorder

Panic disorder is common – 1 in 10 of the population may experience a panic attack at some time in their life. When diagnosing panic disorder, it is important to exclude other causes of the symptoms, such as excessive caffeine, amphetamines or hyperthyroidism.

A cognitive-behavioural approach views panic attacks as *catastrophic misinterpretations of normal bodily symptoms* (Beck, Emery & Greenberg, 1985; Clark, 1986). The patient experiences harmless, often anxiety-related symptoms, and incorrectly interprets them as indicating imminent disaster, such as a heart attack, suffocation or going mad. The anxiety that develops in response to these fears results in further symptoms, such as an increasingly rapid heat beat, dizziness or difficulty concentrating. These symptoms worsen the patient's anxiety and fear as a *vicious cycle*.

Key features of panic attacks:

• They come on suddenly and quickly
• They are associated with intense fear and anxiety
• The most intense feelings of panic are relatively short-lived (although the patient may feel generally anxious to a lesser degree for some time after the most intense feelings have passed)

Thoughts and cognitive factors in panic

During a panic attack, people tend to believe that something *terrible* is about to happen in the very near future. Common fears include going mad, dying or making a fool of themselves in public:

"I am having a heart attack or a stroke."

"I'm going to choke or suffocate."

"I will faint or collapse."

"I am going to lose control."

"I will go mad or crazy."

"I'm going to make a complete fool of myself in front of everyone."

These thoughts may occur as part of a negative *cascade* of thoughts and fears about the meaning of the current situation, with each thought becoming progressively more terrifying:

"*I'm breathing fast.*"

⇓

"*There must be something wrong with me.*"

⇓

"*It's getting more difficult to catch my breath.*"

⇓

"*I must get more air.*"

⇓

"*I can't breathe.*"

⇓

"*I'm going to suffocate and die.*"

Identifying thoughts in anxiety disorders

It is essential to establish what patients feared most *at the time* of the panic attack, rather than their opinion with hindsight, which may be more realistic. Remember that patients may not be consciously aware of the precise nature of their thoughts until they begin to explicitly discuss them.

It is often helpful to use the consultation skill of remaining *specific and concrete*, by asking the patient to describe a typical, recent example of a panicky episode. Then, ask the patient what their exact thoughts and fears were during this experience.

"*What thoughts went through your mind?*"

"*What did you think was happening, or was about to happen to you, at this point?*"

"*What physical symptoms did you notice? What did you think that these might be due to?*"

Patients may be vague when describing thoughts and fears, such as saying, "*Something bad might happen.*" It is important to identify *specific*, negative predictions for the future, such as:

"*I am going to have a heart attack.*"

"*I don't want to go to the party because everyone will ignore me.*"

"*I will make a complete fool of myself by collapsing in front of everyone.*"

In order to identify these specific negative thoughts, the GP can ask questions such as:

"*When you say that* [something bad might happen], *what do you mean?*"

"*What is the worst thing that could happen?*"

"*What is so bad about that?*"

By knowing these predictions, it becomes possible to later test out whether they are true by using techniques to evaluate and reframe thoughts or using behavioural experiments.

Case example 11.1: Identifying thoughts associated with anxiety

Linda is 52 and has been experiencing anxiety with occasional panic attacks over the past six months. She attends her GP, hoping to understand more about why she is getting anxious and how she can learn to manage her feelings of anxiety and panic more easily.

Linda explains that she feels extremely anxious at the thought of going into busy shops, such as supermarkets. In the following dialogue, Linda's GP explores the specific fears that underlie this:

GP You said that you feel anxious at the thought of going into the supermarket. What is it about this situation that makes you feel so anxious?

Linda Well, I might not cope with it.

GP I see. When you say "I might not cope," what do you mean by this?

Linda I mean that I might do become really anxious and make a fool of myself in front of everyone.

GP What do you mean by "make a fool of myself"? What would you do?

Linda If I had a panic attack, it would be really embarrassing.

GP So, having a panic attack might mean that you made a fool of yourself?

Linda Yes.

GP What can you imagine happening during the panic attack that might mean that you made a fool of yourself?

Linda My mind gets confused and my thoughts race so much during the attack. I get scared that I might start babbling complete nonsense to other people. I might lose control and start shouting or making such a scene that other people will think I am completely crazy and I could get taken away to a mental hospital.

GP That sounds like quite a scary image to have in your mind.

Linda Yes, it's really terrifying sometimes.

GP I'm pleased that you were able to share that with me. Maybe we can talk about your fears and try to make that image a bit less frightening.

Linda It would be a huge relief if we were able to do that.

Reminders: Cognitive factors in panic

- During panic attacks, people believe that something *catastrophic* is about to happen in the very near future, such as going mad, dying, or making a fool of themselves in public
- There is often a rapid cascade of increasingly terrifying thoughts and fears about the current situation
- Try to establish what patients most feared *at the time* of the panic attack, by asking them to describe a typical, recent example of a panicky episode
- Identifying *specific*, negative predictions for the future enables these fears to be tested out using cognitive reframing or behavioural experiments

Feelings and emotions in panic disorder

The commonest feelings in panic attacks are extreme anxiety and intense fear. These usually arise suddenly and are usually relatively short-lived. The feelings are extremely distressing and unpleasant.

Physical symptoms/biological reactions in panic

The physical response to panic reflects the adrenaline-based, sympathetic response to fear. This results in a wide variety of powerful and often unpleasant physical symptoms, including:

- Rapid heart beat, palpitations
- Rapid breathing (hyperventilation)
- Feeling short of breath
- Chest pain
- Tightness in the throat, choking sensations
- Gastro-intestinal symptoms: feeling nauseous, abdominal pains
- Feeling faint, dizzy or unsteady
- Numbness and tingling in fingers, toes and lips
- Shaking
- Headache, back pain
- Sweating and hot flushes
- Difficulty concentrating
- Feelings of unreality – as if separated from everything around

The role of behaviour in panic disorder

During a panic attack, people believe strongly that they are threatened by a serious, imminent danger. Their behavioural reactions are therefore usually aimed at preventing this harm from occurring. Common reactions include:

1. *Escape from 'dangerous' situations*

   People commonly react by *escaping* from particular situations that they view as dangerous, perhaps by going home or finding someone with whom they feel safe.

2. *Avoidance*

   Avoidance is a common behavioural reaction associated with nearly all anxiety disorders. Because anxiety is very unpleasant, patients tend to *avoid* situations that they associate with anxiety. This might include avoiding busy shops, confined spaces or particular tasks such as giving presentations. Unfortunately, the long-term effect of avoidance is to make things more difficult for anxious patients, who lose confidence in their ability to deal with stressful situations and become even more anxious. Their lives may become increasingly restricted and they become 'ruled' by their anxiety.

3. *'Safety behaviours'*

Patients often undertake specific actions that make themselves feel safer. They believe that these behaviours can protect them from their most feared outcome. Many of these behaviours become habitual. This might include:

- Resting or avoiding exercise to prevent a heart attack
- Opening windows or breathing deeply to ensure they get enough air and prevent suffocation
- Trying to control their thoughts if they are afraid of going mad
- Seeking medical attention, by calling an ambulance or attending their doctor
- Only going to places with someone else with whom they feel safe
- 'Body scanning' – continually checking their body for symptoms that might indicate imminent disaster

The specific behaviour patterns will depend upon the particular beliefs that the patient holds about the meaning of their symptoms (*Box 11.1*).

Box 11.1: Links between physical sensations, thoughts and behaviour

Sensations	Misinterpretation/thought	Behaviour
Palpitations, racing heart Chest tightness Sweating	*"I'm dying."* *"I'm having a heart attack"*	Sit down, avoid exertion Take medication (e.g. beta-blockers) Try to slow heart rate
Breathless	*"I'm going to suffocate"* *"I can't breathe"* *"I'm choking"*	Take deep breaths Sit by open windows Go into open air
Unreality Muddled thinking Unable to concentrate	*"I might lose control"* *"I'm going mad"* *"Other people will think I'm crazy"*	Try to keep control of mind Look for exits in public Avoid public areas
Dizziness	*"I'm going to faint or collapse"*	Sit down Hold onto someone Avoid going out alone

The effect of unhelpful behaviours in panic disorder

Behavioural reactions often play a key role in maintaining and worsening the feelings of panic as a vicious cycle. Behaviour such as avoidance or escape from frightening situations can prevent the patient from discovering that the feared catastrophe would probably never have happened. Instead, the patient assumes that their behavioural reaction was responsible for keeping them safe (*"If I hadn't left the room at that point then I would have definitely lost control..."*). If the patient remains to face the scary situation, then they are likely to learn that no harm would have come to them and develop confidence that they *can* cope without taking any special precautions.

From Theory to Practice...	Try using the following example to illustrate the unhelpful effect of safety behaviours to patients: *A child believes that a monster lives under her bed. She feels certain that if she were to look under the bed, the monster will leap out and eat her. So, she avoids looking under the bed, and never gets eaten. In the child's mind, this proves that as long as she avoids looking under the bed, she will remain safe.* *How can this child discover that there really is no monster under the bed?*

Some behaviour may actually make things *worse*, by directly *increasing* the intensity of physical symptoms. For example, taking deep breaths when fearing suffocation will increase hyperventilation and its associated symptoms.

Body scanning or continually monitoring and focusing on bodily sensations acts to *increase* the patient's awareness of normal sensations which do not have any sinister significance. Everyone experiences strange bodily sensations from time to time – this might be noticing a pain, becoming aware of our heartbeat or a range of other possibilities. In panic, people become hyper-aware of these normal sensations and then interpret them negatively, which may trigger the panic cycle.

From Theory to Practice...	Use the following experiment to explain the unhelpful effect of concentrating on bodily symptoms to patients: Take a few moments to pay attention to your left foot. Notice any sensations, including temperature, pain, aches or any other physical feelings that may be present. *What sensations did you become aware of? What was the impact of looking for physical feelings?* Most people find that as soon as they begin to look for physical sensations, they become aware of them. Common feelings include tingling, heaviness or discomfort. If we are not concerned about the meaning of such sensations, then noticing them is unlikely to result in anxiety. Imagine, however, if you noticed tingling in your foot and thought to yourself, *"This must mean that I'm having a stroke."* This is very likely to lead to feelings of anxiety, which may be further compounded by *normal* physiological reactions to fear, such as hyperventilation, which further increase sensations of tingling or dizziness and reinforce fears about having a stroke.

Attempts to suppress or control thoughts are likely to paradoxically *increase* the level and intrusive nature of anxious thoughts (see 'Pink elephant experiment', Box 7.2, p. 110).

Asking about behaviour

Always ask anxious patients how they respond behaviourally to anxiety symptoms:

> *"What do you do when you get anxious? How do you react?"*

> *"Is there anything that you are avoiding because it makes you feel anxious?"*

Remember to also ask about the specific thoughts and fears that account for these responses:

> *"What makes you react that way? What might happen if you didn't?"*

> *"What is the worst possible thing that you are trying to avoid?"*

> *"What do you do to try to prevent these fears from coming true?"*

Reminders: The role of behaviour in anxiety and panic

- Avoidance of anxiety-provoking situations lowers people's confidence in their ability to deal with stress and increases long-term anxiety levels
- Safety behaviours prevent people from learning that their perception of danger was exaggerated or inaccurate and reinforce people's fear of certain situations
- Some behaviours, like hyperventilation, make anxiety *worse* by *increasing* the intensity of physical symptoms
- Body scanning causes anxiety by increasing the patient's awareness of normal bodily sensations

---

How do panic attacks arise?

A variety of factors may be involved in the development of panic attacks. Specific triggers for panic might include having an anxiety-provoking automatic thought 'pop' into the mind, becoming aware of particular physical sensations or entering an anxiety-provoking situation. Even when a panic attack seems to arise 'out of the blue', there is still usually a trigger of some kind, though it may be very subtle.

Panic usually arises from misinterpretation of normal bodily sensations. Therefore, anything that alters physical sensations can trigger the panic cycle. Common triggers include:

- Upsetting thoughts or images that result in emotional and physical changes
- Emotional states such as anger, worry or tension
- Physical symptoms related to minor illness
- The effect of drugs, including alcohol or caffeine
- Physical exertion causing changes in heart rate and breathing

Anxiety and panic are common co-existing problems in depressed patients, who may try to ignore or suppress particular worries or negative feelings. These can increase patients' underlying levels of anxiety and tension, eventually resulting in a panic attack. Periods of stress due to social or environmental problems such as financial or relationship difficulties may also contribute to the development of panic attacks. The increased background level of stress and anxiety make it more likely for anxious moments to spiral into panic attacks, when in normal circumstances people would be able to cope with the situation without panicking.

Panic attacks are more likely to arise in people with a pre-existing tendency to concerns about health, and associated beliefs that physical symptoms are likely to indicate something serious. These people are more likely to interpret bodily symptoms as evidence of potentially disastrous consequences. They may develop panic attacks when they develop physical symptoms related to a relatively minor physical disorder, such as a viral illness.

Once the patient has experienced a panic attack, they may develop future anxiety about the possibility of having another one. This panic about panic leads to a vicious cycle.

Vicious cycles in panic disorder

The vicious cycles of panic disorder are illustrated in *Figure 11.1* .

Figure 11.1: CBM of panic – vicious cycles

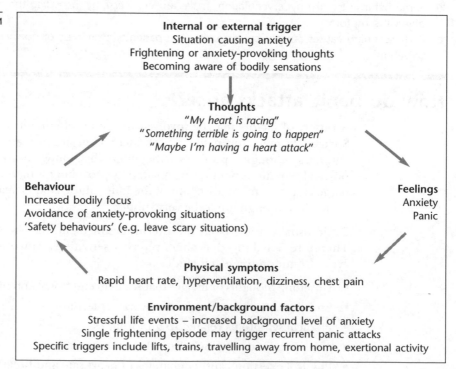

Internal or external trigger
Situation causing anxiety
Frightening or anxiety-provoking thoughts
Becoming aware of bodily sensations

Thoughts
"My heart is racing"
"Something terrible is going to happen"
"Maybe I'm having a heart attack"

Behaviour
Increased bodily focus
Avoidance of anxiety-provoking situations
'Safety behaviours' (e.g. leave scary situations)

Feelings
Anxiety
Panic

Physical symptoms
Rapid heart rate, hyperventilation, dizziness, chest pain

Environment/background factors
Stressful life events – increased background level of anxiety
Single frightening episode may trigger recurrent panic attacks
Specific triggers include lifts, trains, travelling away from home, exertional activity

Managing Anxiety and Panic

Explaining the nature of anxiety

Educating patients about the purpose and nature of anxiety often helps to reduce their fear of experiencing panic attacks. A key aim for managing panic disorder in a patient is to increase their understanding of the nature of panic attacks. This involves helping patients to realize that symptoms simply represent normal physiological responses to scary thoughts and situations, rather than signs of a potentially life-threatening condition.

It is important to reassure patients that panic attacks are not a sign of serious mental illness. The physical sensations that patients experience during panic attacks are *real*. But they arise due to terrifying thoughts and fears, rather than due to imminent physical or psychological disaster.

The purpose of fear and anxiety

Anxiety and fear responses have evolved over millions of years to protect us from physical danger (the *'fight or flight response'*) and are very useful in the right time and place. The symptoms of panic are not a sign that something is going wrong – they merely indicate that the body is doing exactly the right thing to prepare for the perceived threat.

Problems only arise when the fear response is happening at the wrong time or when it persists beyond the point where it is useful. In the modern world, people rarely face physical threats – these physical preparations made by the body may be *unhelpful* in many circumstances, but are *not* dangerous.

Case example 11.2: Explaining the purpose of anxiety responses

---

Priya attends her GP with recurrent anxiety and panic attacks. During a panicky episode, she becomes shaky, sweaty and aware of her heart racing. She finds these experiences terrifying and would like to understand what is happening to her.

In the following dialogue, Priya and her GP discuss her bodily responses during panic attacks:

GP   I'd like to explain a bit more about the body's response to fear and anxiety. Let's use an example:

Imagine you are walking alone along a dark street. You are in a strange town and have got lost. Behind, you hear footsteps and looking back, you see a large man with a hood covering his face. The man follows every turning you make. Although you start to walk more quickly, he begins to get closer. Tell me, how are you feeling in this situation?

continued

Priya I would feel scared.

GP What might you notice physically?

Priya I might have sweaty palms and my heart might beat faster.

GP Right. Now, going back to the scene. You turn another corner, walking faster to try to get away. Suddenly you realize you have turned down a dead end and he has turned in behind you. How do you feel now?

Priya I feel even more frightened. I might be breathing fast and my heart would be really racing.

GP Suddenly the man rushes towards you. He is holding a huge stick. He jumps and tries to grab you. How do you feel now?

Priya I'd be absolutely terrified. I probably wouldn't think very clearly. My heart would be pounding and my chest might feel tight.

GP OK, you have mentioned quite a few physical reactions in this example. You mentioned a racing heart, sweaty palms, breathing fast, having a tight chest and not thinking clearly. Now let's think about *why* you might develop some of these symptoms.

Tell me, how might you get away from this dangerous situation?

Priya I need to get past him and run away.

GP Right, to survive the danger you either need to *run away* or *fight* him. This is known as the *fight or flight response*. It is a natural response of the body to danger, which is controlled by the hormone called adrenaline.

Priya Yes, I've heard of that.

GP So, if you need to be able to run away quickly or fight, will the muscles of your body need more or less fuel?

Priya They would need more fuel.

GP And what kind of fuel does the body use?

Priya Err, well oxygen.

GP Great. How do we get oxygen into the body?

Priya By breathing.

GP So what will need to happen to your breathing to get more oxygen?

Priya I would breathe faster.

GP Yes, *faster* and *deeper* to get more oxygen into the body. Breathing deeply makes the muscles of your chest work extra hard.

Supposing you went to the gym and did an extra hard work out by lifting a heavy weight in your left arm for a long time. How would your arm feel after a while?

Priya It would start to ache.

continued

GP Yes, it would definitely ache, and if you kept going it might really get uncomfortable. How could this tie in with pain in your chest when you are breathing hard and fast?

Priya It's like a workout for your muscles in the chest and they start to ache.

GP Absolutely right. So now we understand why you might breathe fast and why your chest might hurt. Tell me, how does the oxygen from your lungs get around the body to the muscles where it is needed?

Priya It goes around in the blood stream.

GP Exactly. And what makes the blood move around the body?

Priya The heart pumps it around.

GP Right. So, how can your body get oxygen more quickly round the body to the muscles, where you need it to help you run or fight?

Priya The heart beats faster.

GP Yes, by beating *faster* and *harder*. And what might you notice?

Priya I might notice a racing heart or feel it thumping in my chest.

GP Exactly. And, is it a bad thing to be beating fast like that, if you need the extra oxygen in your muscles?

Priya No, it's what the body needs.

GP Exactly, rather than being harmful, it is a natural response, which helps you escape from a very dangerous situation.

  So how could you relate this discussion to your own panic attacks?

Priya It is really interesting to understand why my body reacts the way it does. It doesn't necessarily mean there is something wrong with me.

GP Exactly. This reaction has evolved over millions of years to help us escape from danger. But in modern life, it may be rather an 'over-reaction' by the body. Still, it is not dangerous. It may feel very unpleasant but it doesn't do any harm.

Priya I've never thought of it like that before. The things I feel are not actually dangerous or harmful.

GP That's right. And remember that these unpleasant feelings will not last very long. After a while, the body switches off the response and the reactions will gradually die away.

Remember to use *guided discovery* to involve the patient in an interactive discussion. Other symptoms to discuss include:

Neck/back pain and muscular shaking
Muscles are tensed in preparation to leap quickly into action. This leads to muscular aches, pains and shaking. Ask the patient to tense their arm for up to a minute. Notice the pain and shaking that arises.

continued

Abdominal pains or cramps, diarrhoea, nausea
Gastrointestinal symptoms arise because digestion is slowed to avoid wasting energy that is needed elsewhere. Salivation is also reduced causing a dry mouth and difficulty swallowing.

Having difficulty concentrating/muddled thoughts
Ask the patient to imagine walking down the same dark street, but this time they are focused on listening to loud music playing on a personal stereo. Concentrating on something else makes people less vigilant and at greater risk of being attacked. Therefore, when anxious, the mind constantly flits around checking for danger.

Light-headedness
This is associated with changes in carbon dioxide levels due to hyperventilation. Despite many patients' fears, this does not indicate that they are likely to faint, as blood pressure tends to *rise* rather than drop during anxiety.

Reminders: The purpose of fear and anxiety

- Fear is a normal, automatic response to perceived danger
- This reaction has evolved over millions of years and is designed to increase survival and coping in the face of real, physical danger
- The fear response makes people alert to a threat and prepares them to take action to cope
- When the danger has passed, anxiety will slowly fade away

Anxiety is like a smoke alarm...

Many anxious people believe that their anxiety symptoms are harmful or indicate some serious underlying problem:

"If I keep on feeling so anxious I will probably go mad."

"If I let my heart continue to race so fast, I will certainly have a heart attack."

People often hope to eliminate anxiety altogether in order to feel better. However, this is unrealistic and may reinforce the underlying belief that anxiety is dangerous and should be avoided at all costs.

It is more helpful for patients to aim to become less concerned when anxiety does arise. This has the additional benefit of reducing unpleasant anxiety symptoms by breaking the vicious cycles that often maintain and worsen anxiety. It can be useful to compare the anxiety response to other protective mechanisms, such as car alarms or smoke alarms.

Case example 11.3: Setting realistic goals for managing anxiety

---

Let's return to the example of Priya and her panic attacks. In the following dialogue, Priya's GP discusses why hoping to eliminate anxiety completely might be unhelpful and unrealistic:

GP It can be useful to think about how having anxiety might actually be important and helpful for us. This can make it seem less scary.

Priya Yes, that makes sense.

GP Do you have a smoke alarm at home?

Priya Yes, I do.

GP Why do you have it? What does it do?

Priya Well, the alarm will go off if there is a fire.

GP So it's a warning system to protect you from fire?

Priya Yes, that's right.

GP Tell me, does your smoke alarm ever go off when there *isn't* a fire?

Priya Oh yes, all the time – usually because of burnt toast!

GP Yes, mine is always going off too! But, did that make you throw the smoke alarm in the dustbin?

Priya No, of course not.

GP Why not?

Priya It could save our lives if there were a real fire.

GP Yes, that's right. How do you react when the smoke alarm goes off? Do you immediately call 999 for the fire brigade?

Priya No! I go and have a look and then switch it off.

GP I see. You go and check for a fire, find out what is making the alarm go off, deal with that and then switch the alarm off. Now, how do you think all of this might relate to your feelings of anxiety?

Priya I suppose getting anxious is a bit like warning signal that might be a bit too sensitive. It goes off sometimes when there isn't really a serious problem.

GP Absolutely right. Just like the smoke alarm, it is a very important and useful protective mechanism.

But, we may sometimes get anxious about something that is not really very serious. This is like the smoke alarm reacting to burnt toast.

Priya I see.

continued

> **GP** So, based on the smoke alarm, what is the best way to react to anxiety?
>
> **Priya** To check out what the danger is and then switch it off if there isn't anything too serious.
>
> **GP** That's right. One of the key aims of working with anxiety is to learn how to check what the problem is and then, if there is no danger, to get back to everyday life without it having such a major effect.
>
> **Priya** I see what you mean. But when I feel anxious, I really do feel very bad. The symptoms are so strong.
>
> **GP** Yes, your anxiety alarms bleep very loudly, to alert you to danger. Imagine how it would be if your smoke alarm was 10 times louder – how would that feel?
>
> **Priya** It would be extremely irritating and probably give me a headache!
>
> **GP** Indeed. But just because the alarm is noisy, doesn't mean it is harmful. So, what are the key points you took from this discussion?
>
> **Priya** Anxiety is a bit like a smoke alarm, it is there to warn of possible danger but it sometimes goes off for no reason, like burning the toast. It can be very noisy but isn't necessarily dangerous.

Reminders: Anxiety is like a smoke alarm

■ Panic attacks involve a *normal* response to fear occurring at an inappropriate time or experiencing an overly powerful response to a minor 'danger'

■ The responses are not dangerous in themselves: they are part of a mechanism designed to protect people from potential danger

■ The aim is to make the anxiety response less overpowering and intrusive and for patients to learn how to switch off the anxiety response when necessary

Managing high levels of anxiety

When patients become increasingly anxious or panicky, it becomes very difficult to think clearly or rationally (*Figure 11.2*). It is therefore necessary for patients to have simple techniques of reducing anxiety to more manageable levels before they will be able to rationally evaluate the level of danger and reframe their perspective. This includes techniques such as distraction or controlled breathing .

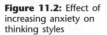

Figure 11.2: Effect of increasing anxiety on thinking styles

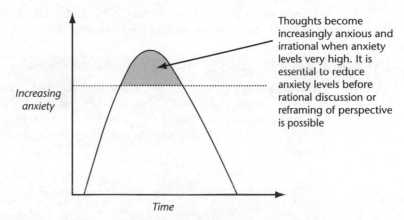

Thoughts become increasingly anxious and irrational when anxiety levels very high. It is essential to reduce anxiety levels before rational discussion or reframing of perspective is possible

Distraction

A simple way to reduce the impact of extremely anxious thoughts and feelings is to use *distraction*. This involves focusing on what is taking place outside or around the patient, rather than focusing on their internal state, which simply increases anxiety. Useful distraction techniques include simple puzzles, mental arithmetic, counting or repeating the words of a song in the mind (see Chapter 7).

Although distraction is a useful short-term strategy for coping with extreme anxiety, remember that it does not help the patient to challenge and overcome their negative thoughts and fears. There is a risk that patients begin to use distraction as a safety behaviour, to avoid facing their fears:

> *"It is dangerous to feel anxious."*
>
> *"If I don't think about things then nothing bad will happen."*
>
> *"If I pay attention to my anxious thoughts then I will become overwhelmed and unable to cope."*

For the long-term, it is also necessary for patients to learn that, whilst *unpleasant*, anxious thoughts and feelings *cannot cause any real harm*.

Relaxation and controlled breathing

Relaxation training can help patients to reduce their background levels of stress and muscular tension, which may reduce the likelihood of developing panic attacks. This could involve practicing techniques such as yoga, progressive muscular relaxation or meditation. Using relaxation tapes or CDs can also be useful (see p. 320 for details). These techniques involve learning a complex *skill*, which needs to be practiced on a regular basis before offering any benefit in reducing panic.

Controlled breathing is a breathing method that helps to avoid hyperventilation and breaks part of the vicious cycle of panic. This technique requires practice when patients are feeling calm and relaxed, before they will be able to use it effectively during panic attacks.

From Theory to Practice...	Here is a method for developing controlled breathing:
	Ask the patient to take a slow, deep breath, whilst counting slowly up to four in their mind. Next, they should hold that in-breath, again counting up to four. Then breathe out slowly, counting slowly to four. Finally, hold the exhaled breath and again count slowly up to four. Thus:
	In 1...2...3...4... Hold 1...2...3...4... Out 1...2...3...4... Hold 1...2...3...4...
	This process should be repeated until they feel more relaxed and calm.
	Ideally, the patient should practice this technique for *four minutes*, carrying it out *four times each day*.

Managing anxious thoughts

A key strategy for managing anxiety disorders is for patients to learn to question the validity of the thoughts that underlie their feelings of anxiety and panic. Patients must learn to view their thoughts as simply thoughts, rather than accurate representations of reality ("*Just because I think I'm having a heart attack doesn't make it true*"). Reducing the number of anxious thoughts can decrease the patient's overall anxiety and reduce the likelihood of their fear spiralling upwards into a panic attack.

Helping patients to view panic as less dangerous

The physical reaction of panic is *self-limiting*. It feels very unpleasant but does not do any real harm and will *always go away after a while*. This fact has

From Theory to Practice...	Ask the patient to count up how many panic attacks they have ever experienced in their life. Be precise by calculating average number per day or week, over a period of months to years. The total number may often be several hundred.
	Ask the patient:
	"*Have you ever actually had a heart attack/gone crazy?*"
	"*Even though you have experienced over 200 panic attacks, nothing has ever actually happened that you really fear. What do you make of this?*"
	Remember to highlight the fact that the feelings of anxiety always go away in the end. If the patient waits long enough, they will feel better. This can be very reassuring for patients to remind themselves during episodes of anxiety.

actually been *proven* in the patient's own experience. The patient has experienced numerous panic attacks, yet the most feared outcome has almost certainly never really occurred.

Dealing with 'what if' thoughts

Thoughts that something terrible is about to happen are common in anxiety disorders, and frequently include *'what if...?'* thoughts. The first step of dealing with these kinds of thoughts is to identify specifically what feared outcomes are being predicted by the patient. This can:

- Help patients to see that their fears are exaggerated and unrealistic
- Enable patients to figure out ways to reduce the chances of the worst outcome actually taking place
- Help the patient to identify how to cope with any difficulties that might arise

Working out ways to cope with feared situations often confers a major sense of relief for patients (*Box 11.2*). This involves taking the mind away from the fear itself and instead focusing on how to cope with it.

Box 11.2: Identifying coping strategies for difficulties

- What skills do you have that might help to deal with this situation?
- What past experiences of similar situations might help you deal with this one?
- What help, advice or support could you obtain available from other people?
- What information could you find out that might help you deal with this situation more effectively?
- Can you change the situation itself, to make things better?
- Can you change the way you *think about* the situation, to make it less stressful?

Another method of coping with 'what if...?' thoughts is to construct a *'then what...?'* plan. This involves identifying the worst possible outcomes and working out a coping strategy to deal with each one.

Case example 11.4: Finding coping strategies for 'what if...?' thoughts

Gabriella is a 22-year old student who suffers from anxiety and occasional panic attacks. She worries a great deal about the problems she faces in her life and experiences many 'what if...?' thoughts which make her feel very anxious.

continued

Next week she has a job interview, which she is extremely nervous about. Her GP helps her to identify coping strategies for her negative, 'what if...?' thoughts, using the questions from Box 11.2:

'What if...?' thoughts/fears	'Then what...?' coping strategy
"What if my mind goes blank during the interview?"	*"I could take a deep breath and tell the interviewers that I feel very nervous and just need a moment to compose myself and then ask them to repeat the question."*
"What if they ask me a question and I can't think of an answer?"	*"I can practice interviews with my friend Claire. She will be able to help me think up ways to answer difficult questions. I will read up on the likely questions that they will ask. If I really don't know the answer then I may have to say so – they might help me out."*
"What if I say something really stupid?"	*"If I realize I have said something stupid then I could say to the interviewer, 'I think I may not have expressed myself very well, what I meant to say was....' Anyway, it's important to remember that it is impossible to be 'perfect' and always say the right thing in an interview."*
"What if they are really aggressive interviewers?"	*"I will try not to take them too seriously. I will just answer the questions as best I can. They will be equally difficult with everyone. I might not even want to work in an office where people are always very aggressive."*
"What if I drop something on my smart clothes before the interview?"	*"I will eat breakfast before I leave home and then not eat anything that could damage my suit once I have left the house. I could also take a small cloth to wipe off anything that I spill."*
"What if I don't get the job?"	*"I can see this interview as good practice for other jobs. I will need to keep applying for jobs until I find the right one."*

Finding evidence for alternative perspectives

It is often useful to look for evidence for and against the most frightening thoughts being accurate. This might involve comparing the evidence for two alternative explanations of the symptoms. It is most helpful if this is done as a *written* thought record. It can also be helpful for patients to write down this evidence onto a 'flashcard', which they can carry around with them and read whenever they feel anxious.

Case example 11.5: Reframing scary thoughts

Peter is 35 years old and has been experiencing panic attacks for the past six months. At the peak of his panic attacks he has the following hot thought: *"If I carry on feeling so bad, then I will have a heart attack."*

Anxious thought to test out:

"If I carry on feeling so bad, then I will certainly have a heart attack."

Evidence *for* hot thought	Evidence *against* the hot thought
What makes you say that this thought is true? Has anything happened to prove it to you? Do any past experiences fit this belief?	Is there anything that shows that the thought is not completely accurate? Are there any other ways to view the situation? Is this way of thinking an 'unhelpful thinking style'? What would be more realistic?
"My heart is racing and I feel sweaty – this is what happens during a heart attack."	*"Having a racing heart and getting sweaty happens for many reasons other than having a heart attack, e.g. during exercise. Exercise is good for the heart."*
"I get chest pain when I feel very anxious – this could be a sign of strain on the heart."	*"Lots of people experience extreme stress, such as being mugged on the street or being a soldier in battle, but don't all have heart attacks."*
"I saw a TV programme where a very stressed-out, anxious man ended up having a heart attack."	*"The anxiety response is a survival mechanism designed to protect me from danger – the 'fight or flight' response. This isn't dangerous – it is a normal, healthy reaction to stressful situations."*
"Anxiety makes my blood pressure go up – this is bad for the heart."	*"I have had many panic attacks and nothing bad has ever actually happened."*
"I feel so bad during the attack – it must be something really serious."	*"I had my heart checked out by the doctor and they found nothing wrong."*
	"Panic does cause a brief rise in my blood pressure but my body is designed to cope with this. It is only if blood pressure is constantly raised that it becomes a problem. My blood pressure has been checked and it is normal."
	"I do feel really bad during panic attacks but this doesn't automatically mean that I am having a heart attack. People can still feel very bad, even when there is no danger, e.g. a child being terrified of a monster in the cupboard."

continued

> **Alternative/balanced thought to replace the hot thought:**
>
> Write an alternative or balanced thought which takes into account evidence for and against the hot thought. Try to be fair and realistic.
> *"The symptoms that I get during a panic attack can be more easily explained by anxiety rather than having a heart attack. They feel really bad but are not dangerous and cannot actually hurt me."*

Reminders: Coping with anxious thoughts and feelings

- Distraction is a useful short-term strategy for managing extreme anxiety, which helps patients to focus on their external, rather than internal environment
- Relaxation and controlled breathing may also be helpful
- Counting how many panic attacks a patient has ever experienced without coming to major harm lends weight to the view that anxiety is not really dangerous
- Dealing with anxious predictions and 'what if...?' thoughts involves constructing a 'then what...?' plan, which identifies coping strategies to deal with potential, future difficulties
- Unrealistic, anxious thoughts can be evaluated using a written thought record to find evidence for alternative explanations for unpleasant, anxiety-related symptoms

Changing unhelpful behaviour in panic disorder

Useful behavioural experiments for anxiety disorders involve finding ways to overcome unhelpful responses such as avoidance or safety behaviour. This includes limiting the use of 'as required' anxiety-reducing medication, such as beta-blockers or benzodiazepines. Whilst this may be a useful strategy in some cases, it is generally more helpful to prescribe medication *regularly*.

Setting up a behavioural experiment involves finding out what happens when the patient faces their fears or stops using certain safety behaviours. This is similar to the child choosing to look under her bed, which is likely to prove that there really is no monster there.

Changing avoidance behaviour

Difficulties should be overcome *gradually* by facing anxiety-provoking situations in easy stages. By practicing easier things first, the patient will develop the confidence to move onto more challenging situations.

It is often helpful to develop a *hierarchy* of scary situations, aiming to gradually work upwards through the list, overcoming each feared situation in turn. Patients can control how quickly they proceed through the list of challenges and should not feel pressurized to proceed more quickly than they feel comfortable with.

There are several stages for using 'graded practice' to overcome avoidance (Kennerley, 1997):

1. Make a list of situations which the patient is avoiding or that make them anxious. Identify a wide range of situations, including several which are not too challenging or frightening

2. Ask the patient to rank the situations into order of increasing difficulty

3. Choose the first situation as a target for the patient to achieve; if it still seems overwhelming, try breaking it down into smaller 'chunks'

4. Work out the key strategies for coping with any difficulties or anxiety that may arise. This might include using distraction, controlled breathing, relaxation or finding alternative perspectives for anxiety-provoking thoughts that are likely to arise

5. The patient tries out the task. They should repeat it several times, until it no longer seems difficult or anxiety-provoking

It can be useful for some patients to work through particularly scary situations in their *imagination*, before trying them out in real life. This involves visualizing themselves successfully coping with the difficulty, including imagining themselves using effective coping strategies to overcome their fear of the situation. This exercise should be repeated several times until the anxiety has reduced and the patient feels ready to try it in reality.

It is common for patients to feel anxious during these types of behavioural experiment. Remind them that anxiety is a normal, healthy emotion, which is not dangerous. The initial aim is not to complete the task *without* anxiety, but to achieve it *despite feeling anxious*. By repeating the task several times, anxiety will naturally reduce over the long-term.

Case example 11.6: Addressing agoraphobia

Beryl suffers from agoraphobia. She experiences anxiety when away from home, especially in busy or crowded areas. This is having a major impact on her life by limiting what she feels able to do each day. She has markedly reduced her social interactions and become depressed.

Beryl's GP explains the rationale for *facing* fears, rather than avoiding them. Together, Beryl and her GP create the following list of anxiety-provoking situations, beginning with the least difficult:

1. Going to the local shop with my husband during a quiet time
2. Going to the local shop and husband waits outside
3. Going to the local shop alone at a quiet time
4. Going to the local shop at a busy time, buying only one or two items
5. Going to the local shop at a busy time and spending longer there, looking for several items
6. Going to a mini-market with my husband
7. Going to the mini-market alone at a quiet time
8. Going to the mini-market alone at a busy time
9. Going to the supermarket at a quiet time

continued

10.   Going to the supermarket at a busy time

Notice how simple tasks like going to the local shop can be broken down into very small stages, which are much less threatening.

Beryl is keen to feel more 'normal' and re-build her life to include activities like shopping. Other graded tasks might involve increasing social activity, enjoyable activities or anything that patients identify as being *important* and *relevant* to their life goals.

Eliciting frightening bodily sensations

In treating panic disorder, it is common to use behavioural experiments which deliberately try to elicit physical sensations that are similar to those experienced by the patient during a panic attack. Through these experiments, the patient learns that the symptoms may be harmless and do not necessarily indicate that a catastrophic outcome is imminent.

This includes experiments such as:

1. *Hyperventilation*

   Breathing deeply and rapidly for a few minutes can produce a wide range of sensations, which may be similar to those experienced during panic. It is a powerful means of producing feelings such as dizziness, faintness, racing heart and paradoxical breathlessness. To enhance learning from this process, it is useful to ask the patient a variety of 'synthesizing' questions:

   "Were these symptoms similar to the ones that occur during panic? What do you make of the fact that you can bring them on, by breathing quickly for a few minutes?"

   "How does this affect the idea that the symptoms mean you are having a heart attack?"

   "Can heart attacks be brought on just by breathing quickly?"

   "How quickly did the symptoms subside after you stopped breathing? What do you make of this?"

   Contraindications to hyperventilation: cardiac problems, high blood pressure, pregnancy and asthma/COPD.

2. *Exercise tasks*

   Some patients avoid exercise due to fears that the associated rapid heart rate or sweating may be dangerous. Challenging these beliefs might involve encouraging the patient to walk quickly up and down steps, skipping, walking briskly or jogging.

3. *Chest pain*

   The patient can be asked to take a deep breath of air and then, whilst holding as much air in as possible, try to continue to breathe forcibly. This often causes some chest discomfort and can be used to reinforce the explanation that chest pain often relates to overuse of thoracic muscles during over-breathing.

4. *'Going crazy'*

For patients who fear 'going crazy' during panic, they could be 'challenged' to make this happen, simply by thinking 'crazy' or uncontrolled thoughts. This can help to reinforce the belief that muddled thinking is a normal part of anxiety and does not necessarily indicate severe mental illness.

Reminders: Changing unhelpful behaviour in anxiety and panic

■ Facing anxiety-provoking situations in gradual stages helps the patient develop confidence to tackle more challenging situations
■ The patient should plan in advance how to cope with any anxiety that may arise
■ It may be necessary for patients to practice facing scary situations in their imagination before trying in real life
■ It is normal to feel anxious during these experiments but this will reduce with practice
■ Behavioural experiments such as hyperventilation are used to challenge beliefs about the meaning of physical symptoms that arise during panic attacks

Box 11.3:
Summary of self-help strategies for managing panic reactions

- Remind yourself that the feelings of panic are *normal bodily sensations* related to anxiety and are not harmful.
- Remember that anxiety, whilst extremely unpleasant, is *not really dangerous*. It is a mechanism which has evolved over millions of years to *protect us* by helping us cope with physical danger.
- Try not to run away. Instead, try to accept what is happening to you. If you wait long enough, the fear will pass. This will make it less likely to arise in the future.
- Use coping strategies like distraction or controlled breathing to reduce your unpleasant anxiety symptoms.
- Remember that frightening thoughts are just *thoughts* – they are not necessarily true or accurate. Just because something *seems true* does not mean that it is.
- Try to find more helpful and realistic ways to look at any thoughts that might be making your anxiety worse.
- When you feel better, think back to what triggered off the panic. What kinds of anxious thoughts were going through your mind? Whilst feeling calmer, try to find a more balanced or way to look at the situation, which might be less likely to make you panic in future.

Chapter 12

Depression

- Depression is common and widespread in primary care settings

- CBT is the most effective psychological treatment for depression

- The CBM offers a useful approach for patients with mild to moderate depression in primary care and can be used as an adjunct to treatments such as medication

- Depression is characterized by negative thoughts about the self, others and the future and by withdrawal from social interaction and reduction of activity

- Behavioural changes such as increasing activity levels are particularly effective for improving depression

Understanding Depression

Depression is common. Between 5 and 10% of people seen in primary care suffer from major depression and as many as 2–3 times more people may experience depressive symptoms but do not meet diagnostic criteria for major depressive disorder (Katon & Schulberg, 1992).

Depression is characterized by persistent low mood, loss of interest and enjoyment in usual activities and reduced energy. These symptoms must be present for at least two weeks and be associated with a marked impairment in daily functioning in order to make a diagnosis of major depression (*Box 12.1*).

Box 12.1:
Diagnosis of major depression (DSM-IV Criteria: APA, 1994)

Five of the following criteria (including at least one of the first two criteria) must have been present *almost every day for more than two weeks*. These features must cause significant impairment in social, occupational or other important areas of functioning.

- Depressed mood for most of the day
- Reduced pleasure or interest in usual activities for most of the day
- Fatigue or loss of energy
- Substantial change in appetite or unintentional weight loss or gain (≥5% of body weight per month)
- Insomnia or hypersomnia
- Psychomotor agitation or retardation
- Diminished ability to think or concentrate, or indecisiveness
- Feelings of excessive guilt or worthlessness
- Recurrent thoughts of death or suicide

The disorder must not be caused by:
- Bereavement
- Organic disease

Recognition of depression

GPs must identify patients with depression, if they are to offer effective treatment for it. However, only about half of depressed people in the community will ever present to their GP and of those patients who do attend, up to 50% of cases are missed (Kessler *et al.*, 1999).

Making a diagnosis in primary care can be tricky – at least two-thirds of depressed people present with physical or somatic rather than psychological symptoms (NICE, 2004b). In patients with co-existing physical disease, making a diagnosis of depression is even less likely, because health professionals tend to focus on physical or somatic symptoms rather than psychological or emotional difficulties (Thompson *et al.*, 2000).

Recognition of depression in primary care can be improved by asking two simple screening questions (*Box 12.2*).

Box 12.2:
Useful screening
questions for
depression

> *"During the last month, have you often been bothered by:*
>
> * *Feeling down, depressed or hopeless?*
> * *Having little interest or pleasure in doing things?"*

A GP's recognition of depression can also be improved by training in effective consultation skills (Moral *et al.*, 2001). Increasing confidence and skills in understanding depression using the CBM is also likely to enhance the GP's ability to detect and manage depressed patients.

Reminders: Recognizing depression

- Depression is common in primary care settings but up to half of cases may be missed
- Depressed patients may present with somatic or physical complaints
- Recognition of depression can be improved by asking two screening questions
- Diagnosis may also be enhanced by improving a GP's consulting style

CBT for depression

CBT is the psychological treatment of choice for depression (NICE, 2004b). It is as effective as antidepressant drug therapy for major depression in primary care (Scott *et al.*, 1997). It also has a lower rate of long-term relapse than antidepressants (Paykel *et al.*, 1999), because patients develop lasting skills in coping with life's inevitable difficulties. In severe depression, a combination of CBT and antidepressants is more effective than either treatment alone.

Many patients prefer psychological approaches for depression. Some patients are sceptical about the benefits of medication and may feel 'fobbed off' if antidepressants are prescribed too readily (Kadam *et al.*, 2001). As many as two-thirds of patients may also believe, mistakenly, that antidepressant medications are addictive (Churchill *et al.*, 2000).

These negative beliefs about medication have been amplified by an increasingly negative media portrayal of antidepressants as dangerous, addictive and inappropriately over-prescribed by GPs. It is therefore important to discuss *all* treatment options with depressed patients, enabling them to make informed decisions about treatments.

A combined approach to depression for primary care

While there is little doubt of the effectiveness of CBT for the management of depression, at present, access to CBT services remains extremely limited in many regions of the UK. A realistic and practical method of managing depression in primary care should therefore include both psychological approaches and medication.

NICE advocates a stepped care approach to depression management (Box 12.3). The first step involves the recognition and assessment of depression, including assessing for suicidal thoughts or intent. The appropriate management depends on the severity of depression. Subsequent steps might involve guided self-help, exercise, antidepressant medication, psychological therapies and the involvement of mental health services where appropriate.

Box 12.3: NICE guidelines for depression (2004b)

	Who is responsible?	What is the focus?	What do they do?
Step 1 Recognition of depression	GP, practice nurse	Recognition of depression	Assessment
Step 2 Treatment of mild depression in primary care	Primary health care team, primary care mental health worker	Mild depression	Watchful waiting, guided self-help, computerized CBT, exercise, brief psychological interventions
Step 3 Treatment of moderate–severe depression in primary care	Primary health care team, primary care mental health worker	Moderate or severe depression	Medication, psychological interventions, social support
Step 4 Treatment by mental health specialists	Mental health specialists including crisis teams	Treatment-resistant, recurrent, atypical and psychotic depression and those at significant risk	Medication, complex psychological interventions, combined treatments
Step 5 In-patient treatment	Inpatient care, crisis teams	Risk to life, severe self-neglect	Medication, combined treatments, ECT

The CBM can be easily incorporated into a GP's existing approaches to the diagnosis and management of depression. It is particularly useful for patients with mild depression, for whom there is little evidence that antidepressant medication is effective. The approach can be combined with self-help strategies and exercise programmes. It may be particularly important when access to standard CBT services is limited.

Reminders: Management of depression

■ CBT is as effective as antidepressant medication for moderate to severe depression with less long-term relapse
■ Many patients prefer psychological therapies to antidepressant medication for depression
■ The CBM is particularly useful for management of mild to moderate depression in primary care
■ The approach can be combined with self-help, exercise and antidepressant medication

Aetiology of depression

Risk factors for depression include a variety of biological, psychological and social factors (*Box 12.4*). Biological factors include inherited tendencies to depression. However, although there is an increased risk of depression in the children of depressed parents, its development is not *inevitable* and depends on a variety of other psychological and social factors.

Psychological factors associated with depression include negative life events, particularly during childhood and early life. The loss of a parent or the experience of childhood abuse may leave people more vulnerable to developing depression in later life. Ongoing social difficulties such as financial problems, poor housing or lack of social support, which lead to chronic stress, are also associated with depression.

The development of depression usually depends on a combination of factors, which may be related. For example, if someone experiences the early loss of a parent, they may develop depression when faced by loss or bereavement in later life.

Box 12.4: Risk factors for depression

- Female sex: women are twice as likely to develop depression, particularly if caring for young children and lacking social support
- Unemployment
- Family history of depression
- Loss of a parent before adolescence
- Lack of social support network (e.g. close friends or family)
- Experiencing multiple negative life events
- Presence of chronic physical disorders

Reminders: Aetiology of depression

■ Biological, psychological and social factors play a role in the aetiology of depression.
■ Depression is never *inevitable* – its development depends on the complex interaction of these factors

Features of depression

CBT takes a holistic approach to understanding depression in terms of the interaction between psychological factors (how people think and cope in various situations), biological and bodily processes, and social, cultural and economic circumstances, including early life experiences and current life events (*Figure 12.1*).

Figure 12.1:
Summary of the
CBM for depression

Thoughts/thinking styles	Feelings
Negative thoughts: self-criticism, negative view of world, hopelessness Low motivation	Sadness, low mood Loss of enjoyment Anxiety Guilt, shame, anger

Behaviour	Physical symptoms
Reduce enjoyable and meaningful activities Avoid social interaction Excessive rest Other unhelpful activities, e.g. misuse alcohol/drugs, self-harm, reassurance-seeking	Low energy and tiredness Poor concentration and memory Disturbed sleep Changes in appetite and weight

Environment/social factors
Lack of social support
Unemployment
Family history of depression
Loss of a parent before adolescence
Experiencing negative life events

Cognitive aspects of depression

Depressed people characteristically develop *negative* thinking styles, which includes negative thoughts about themselves (self-criticism), about the world and about the future (hopelessness). These thoughts are often examples of *unhelpful thinking styles* (*Box 12.5*).

Box 12.5:
Common
unhelpful
thinking styles
in depression

- Black-and-white thinking (*"I am completely useless"*)
- Negative, self-critical view of self (*"I am such an idiot"*)
- Ignoring positives (*"Nothing went well this week"*)
- Mind-reading (*"He thought I was boring"*)
- Negative view of the future (*"Nothing will ever get any better"*) and predicting catastrophes
- Taking excessive personal responsibility/self-blame (*"I ruined the party for everyone"*)

1. Negative thoughts about self

Self-critical and self-blaming thoughts are very common in depression:

"I'm a terrible parent."

"I lost the job because I'm useless."

"I'm a burden to others."

"I'm no good at anything."

These thoughts are damaging because they lower confidence, reduce self-esteem and cause problems in relationships with others. They are also *self-fulfilling* because thinking so negatively is likely to prevent people from behaving in constructive or positive ways.

2. *Negative thoughts about the world*

Depressed people tend to take a negative and pessimistic view of the world. They often misinterpret events by jumping to the worst conclusions, and perceive others as critical, uncaring or hurtful. Focusing on one minor criticism whilst ignoring a barrage of compliments is another example of negative thinking about the world.

"The world is so full of terrible events – everything is just pointless."

"Nothing ever goes right for me."

"Nobody likes me."

"That waiter was rude because he did not respect me."

3. *Negative thoughts about the future*

Negative thinking or hopelessness about the future is particularly important in depression. Predicting that the future is bleak and that nothing will ever improve is likely to make patients feel disheartened and despondent. At its most severe, hopelessness can be linked with suicidal thoughts and behaviour.

"Nothing good will ever happen to me."

"I'll never get a job – what's the point in trying?"

"I will never get over this depression. Nothing will get any better."

Case example 12.1: Identifying negative thoughts in depression

Cathy is a 26-year old bank clerk who suffers from mild depression. Here, she describes a barbecue that she attended at the weekend:

"I went to Alison's barbeque at the weekend. I didn't really want to go, because I knew that I wouldn't really enjoy it. I never have anything interesting to say. While I was there I made a terrible mistake – I forgot the name of Alison's sister, Joanne. I've only met her a couple of times before and my mind went blank. I was so embarrassed. I looked like a complete fool. I'm sure Joanne was really offended. I tried to make it up to her by apologizing and asking about her children, but I don't think that was enough. Alison will never invite me to any more parties."

Read through the text and identify Cathy's negative or unhelpful thoughts:

continued

> *Negative, unhelpful thoughts:*
> I won't enjoy the barbecue
> I never have anything interesting to say
> I made a terrible mistake by forgetting Joanne's name
> I looked like a complete fool
> Joanne was really offended
> Alison will never invite me to any more parties
> *Which unhelpful thinking styles are represented by these thoughts (see Box 12.5 for a reminder)?*

Reminders: Cognitive aspects of depression

■ Depressed people have negative, unhelpful thoughts about themselves, the world and the future
■ Highly self-critical thoughts damage confidence and self-esteem
■ Negative thoughts are often self-fulfilling and worsen depressed moods
■ Hopelessness involves a highly negative view of the future and can be associated with suicidal thoughts and behaviour

From Theory to Practice...	Notice the negative thoughts displayed by depressed people. Look for negative thoughts about the self, world and future. Which unhelpful thinking styles are most common?
	At this stage, do not attempt to *challenge* these thoughts. Simply highlight their presence to the patient and discuss the impact of thinking so negatively.

Feelings and emotions in depression

Depressed people experience a wide variety of negative emotions. These include:

• Persistent depressed mood – includes feeling sad, low, bleak, numb and empty

• Loss of enjoyment or pleasure in usual activities

• Anxiety, tension and panic

• Anger and irritability: with self and others

• Guilt and self-blame

• Shame – relating to perceived inferiority to others or failure

Biological factors and physical symptoms in depression

Depression is associated with a wide range of unpleasant physical feelings and symptoms. These include:

- *Low energy and lethargy:* feeling tired all the time – results in reduced activity levels
- *Disturbed sleep:* includes difficulty getting off to sleep, early morning wakening or excessive sleeping
- *Difficulty concentrating:* people may find it difficult to read or follow a TV programme or conversation
- *Memory problems:* short-term memory becomes poor because of difficulties concentrating. People may also selectively remember negative events
- *Changes in appetite and weight:* usually a loss of appetite and weight, but some people may 'comfort eat' and gain weight
- *Reduced libido:* loss of interest in sex
- *Becoming 'slowed up' (psycho-motor retardation):* people often think and move more slowly than usual. This may include other bodily functions such as becoming constipated
- *Physical agitation:* increased muscular tension and restlessness
- *Increased pain:* people often feel pain more intensely when depressed
- *Associated physical conditions:* people may have greater difficulty coping with existing physical disorders or may develop new conditions such as headaches or irritable bowel syndrome.

Understanding that all of these physical problems may relate to depression can be a major relief for depressed people, who often fear that each symptom indicates an independent, major problem. Many of these symptoms resolve when the underlying depression lifts, although it can sometimes be useful to address particularly troublesome symptoms, such as severe insomnia, individually.

Biological changes in depression also include changes in levels of neurotransmitters in the brain, such as serotonin, dopamine and noradrenaline. This causes alterations in brain function, including reduced positive emotions and changes in sleep, appetite and motivation. Antidepressants improve depression by boosting the levels of these neurotransmitters.

From Theory to Practice...	Remember to ask depressed people about any physical symptoms, including low energy and fatigue, that they are experiencing. It can be reassuring for the patient to realize that these symptoms are related to their depression.

Reminders: Physical and biological changes in depression

■ Depression is associated with a range of unpleasant physical symptoms, which patients may not directly link to depression

■ Low energy and tiredness are common and result in reduced activity levels

■ Other physical changes include poor sleep, changes in appetite and weight, difficulty concentrating and increased pain.

Altered behaviour in depression

Unhelpful behaviour plays a key role in or maintaining feelings of depression. This includes:

1. Reduced activity

Depressed people tend to withdraw from social activity. They reduce participation in enjoyable activities, such as meeting friends or pursuing hobbies and interests, and may only carry out essential jobs which are less interesting or fun.

Depressed people may also reduce activities that give life a sense of meaning or achievement, such as taking exercise, going to work or daily activities like household chores. In more severe depression, people reduce self-care. They may wash less frequently, pay less attention to appearance or clothes, forget to shave or brush their hair, and eat badly.

These changes in behaviour may be due to:

- Lethargy and tiredness *("I'm too tired – I don't have enough energy")*
- Depressed mood and lack of enjoyment in usual activities *("There's no point in going because I don't enjoy anything these days")*
- Negative thinking and low motivation *("I can't be bothered to try")*

Reducing enjoyable activities heightens people's feelings of depression and despair because life becomes increasingly mundane and isolated. Avoiding routine tasks and chores, such as ironing or washing up, can make people feel ashamed and guilty, and increases their sense of failure and lack of worth *("I can't even manage to keep the house tidy – I'm completely useless")*.

2. Increased unhelpful activities

Depressed patients may also develop new, unhelpful behaviours, which make their problems worse, including:

- Excessive rest and over-sleeping (which exacerbates lethargy)
- Misuse of alcohol or drugs
- Self-harm
- Making excessive demands or seeking reassurance from others
- Sabotaging their own attempts to achieve positive goals ('setting themselves up to fail')
- Behaving in ways which increases the likelihood of being let down or rejected by others

Reminders: Behaviour changes in depression

■ Depressed people often withdraw from social interaction and reduce pleasurable activities

■ Excessive rest and oversleeping acts to increase lethargy and fatigue further

■ Other unhelpful behaviour includes misuse of alcohol/drugs, reassurance-seeking, self-harm or 'setting themselves up to fail'

From Theory to Practice...	Ask depressed patients whether they are behaving differently: *"What do you do differently, now that you feel so depressed? How did you behave before you felt depressed?"* Is this behaviour helpful or unhelpful? How does it affect their depressed feelings?

The role of environmental and social factors in depression

Life events, social difficulties and environmental problems, both past and present, all contribute to the development of depression.

When faced by a large number of difficulties, people may feel overwhelmed and become depressed. It is important to spend time reviewing any key environmental and social factors which contribute to the development and maintenance of depression in any individual.

Vicious cycles in depression

Relationships between negative thoughts and feelings

Negative thoughts and feelings are closely linked. Negative thinking results in feeling more depressed. Equally, feeling low is also likely to generate a host of negative thoughts and reflections.

Negative thoughts
"I am boring and unattractive"
"Nobody likes me"

Depressed mood
Sad and low

Reducing activity

Reducing activity levels, particularly those which are enjoyable or which give life a sense of meaning or achievement, makes depressed people feel even worse:

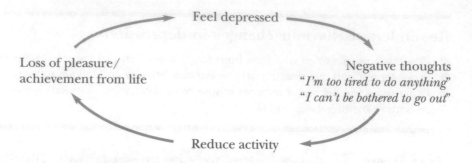

Withdrawal from social interaction

By withdrawing from contact with other people, depressed people become increasingly isolated and lonely. They may repeatedly refuse invitations or behave in a withdrawn manner, such as by avoiding eye contact or speaking to others. Consequently, other people stop offering invitations to social events, assuming that the depressed person does not wish to be invited, or even that the depressed person does not like *them*. This makes life feel even more isolated and empty.

The influence of lethargy and tiredness

Depressed people commonly feel tired and lethargic. This tends to reduce activity even further.

A vicious cycle arises because the tiredness associated with depression is *made worse* by rest. This is similar to the strong feelings of drowsiness or lethargy that often arise after a daytime nap. It is useful to explain this counterintuitive fact to patients.

The most helpful and effective way to increase energy and reduce tiredness in depression is to *increase activity*. This energizes and awakens people, frequently improving their feelings and mood.

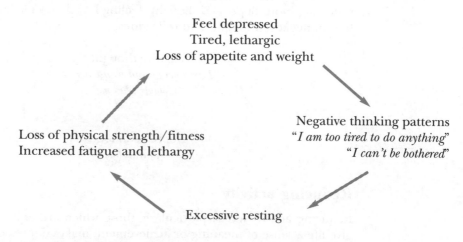

Reminders: Vicious cycles in depression

- Reducing activity levels, particularly enjoyable activities, makes depressed people feel worse
- Social withdrawal makes depressed people more isolated, lonely and unhappy
- Excessive rest *increases* tiredness rather than alleviating it – increasing activity is the best way to boost energy and improve mood

From Theory to Practice...	Remember to gather information about all five areas of the CBM when assessing depressed patients. Make particular note of any unhelpful behaviour such as reducing activity. Can you identify any vicious cycles? What might be the easiest way to break these?

Approaches to Overcoming Depression

Working through the CBM with depressed patients

Making effective use of the CBM with depressed patients

Depressed people usually welcome a psychological approach to their problems, but there are some difficulties in using the model with this group. Problems such as tiredness, lethargy, difficulty concentrating and a continual barrage of self-critical, negative thoughts will make it difficult for depressed people to actively engage in the hard work required to use cognitive-behavioural approaches effectively.

These obstacles can be addressed directly using basic principles of the CBM. For example, thoughts, such as *"This will never help me, there is no point in trying. I will never get better,"* can be used as examples of negative, unhelpful thinking styles that can be challenged and re-framed.

There are some key consultation skills that GPs can use to help patients overcome these difficulties (*Box 12.6*).

Box 12.6: Key consultation skills to use with depression	• *Written information:* this is especially important in depression where patients have poor concentration and memory. Consider offering a video or audio-recording of the consultation for them to review at home • *Cognitive empathy:* be interested in explore the *meaning* of difficult situations for individual patients

- *Focus on specific, concrete examples:* This helps avoid becoming overwhelmed by patients' multiple, complex problems. Ask the patient to choose the most important issue to discuss
- *Guided discovery:* encourage patients to take the lead in discussions and discover new perspectives for situations *themselves*. Remember that depressed people may think slowly and have difficulty concentrating. Keep questions simple and allow them time to come up with answers
- *Homework*: encourage the patient to make real changes in their life based on the information gathered by the CBM. Focus on increasing activity levels. Remember to review homework when you next see the patient

Case example 12.2: Using the CBM to understand depressed patients

The following example shows how the CBM can be used to understand depressed patients. Read through the dialogue and try to break down Roger's problems into the five areas of the CBM.

Background:
Roger is a 40-year old English teacher who has been depressed on and off for two years. His wife is also a teacher and is very supportive. His GP has known him for about a year. Roger became more depressed six months ago, when he was having problems with a colleague at work. He started antidepressant medication, which did improve his mood and had few side effects. However, he still periodically feels low and depressed. He attends the surgery for a repeat prescription of his medication. He is also hoping to discuss his progress with his GP:

Roger I'm taking the tablets and they are helping. I feel better than before. I don't want to change my medication, but I do still sometimes feel very low. I feel stuck as I would like to on with life and stop feeling so down.
GP Have you any thoughts as to what you would like to try?
Roger I'm really not sure.
GP There are ways to help people feel more positive and improve depression that do not involve changing medication. Would you like to discuss these possibilities?
Roger Yes, I think that would be helpful.
GP Perhaps we could start by getting an understanding of your difficulties. What is bothering you most at the moment?
Roger I'm an English teacher. I enjoy teaching the children but I have a lot of difficulty during staff meetings. You may remember the

continued

problems I had with my previous head of department – she was a real bully. She has left now but I still feel very anxious and lack confidence in meetings. I also feel quite tired a lot of the time, so I can't get much done. I keep putting off jobs like marking or lesson planning, so it's constantly building up and causing me stress. And my social life is awful – I just don't really get out very much at all.

GP I see. It sounds like there are several different aspects to your difficulties. You mentioned problems during staff meetings, feeling tired, putting off jobs like marking and not having a great social life. What would be the most helpful area to focus on first?

Roger One of the worst things is that I can't seem to keep up with jobs like marking or writing reports. They build up and I feel really anxious about it. Eventually, they become such a huge job, I can't even face starting.

GP Perhaps we could write down what you say in the form of this chart, which is broken down into different areas: thoughts, feelings, physical symptoms, behaviour and other issues in your environment. This might help show some patterns and find ways to improve matters. Does that seem OK with you?

Roger I'm not quite sure what you mean by some of those things.

GP I hope it will make more sense as we work through. Firstly, can you think of a recent example of a time when you were struggling with doing some marking or writing reports?

Roger Yes, only last night, I had a big pile of books to mark but I didn't get around to it.

GP OK, that's a good start. How did you feel about having all that marking to do?

Roger I felt really depressed. I felt like I wouldn't ever be able to cope with the workload.

GP [*Writing down relevant info*] I see. At what point in the evening did you feel the worst?

Roger As soon as I got home and realized I had all that work to do, I started feeling low and I stayed that way all evening.

GP Oh dear, that sounds very unpleasant. Let me check that I understood you correctly. You said that you were feeling depressed and low and thinking *'I will never cope with all this workload'*. Is that correct?

Roger Yes it is.

GP What else was going through your mind?

Roger I didn't think I could manage it – it all seemed too complicated. I kept thinking I would probably make a mess of things.

GP Right, you thought *'I can't manage this – it's too complicated and I will probably make a mess of things.'* What else stopped you from getting on with the work?

Roger I just felt too tired and sluggish.

GP So how did you react when you were feeling that way? What did you do that evening?

continued

Roger I just ignored the work and dozed in front of the TV all evening.

GP Tell me, how did you feel after that?

Roger I felt really fed up that I hadn't achieved anything. It means I'm really a terrible teacher.

GP And did you feel more energetic after resting for the whole evening?

Roger No, I felt really sleepy and exhausted.

GP OK, that is all really interesting information. Let's have a look at what you said...

Roger's CBM chart:

Situation: Tuesday evening, coming home from school and realizing there is huge amount of marking to do.

Thoughts	Feelings
"I won't ever be able to cope with this workload – there's too much to do." *"I can't manage this – I will just make a mess of it."* *"I haven't achieved anything this evening"* *"I'm a terrible teacher."*	Depressed Down Fed up
Behaviour	**Physical symptoms**
Puts off starting the work Rests/dozes on the sofa all evening	Tired and sluggish Sleepy and exhausted

Environment/situation/other problems
Works as English teacher in a secondary school Married to Valerie, no children, good relationship Problems last year with a difficult boss – little confidence in own work Lack of social life

The CBM approach to overcoming depression

A key aim of using the CBM is to enable the patient to understand depression better. Using the CBM to 'map out' and explain depression may help patients to identify ways of improving their problems.

Remember to use 'synthesizing' questions to encourage the patient to reflect on their experience of depression in the light of the new information gathered by using the CBM approach, such as:

"What do you make of all this information that we have gathered?"

"How could you use this approach to help you improve things?"

There is a variety of useful cognitive-behavioural strategies for improving depression (*Box 12.7*).

Box 12.7:
Cognitive-
behavioural
treatment
strategies for
depression

- Behavioural activation – increasing activities boosts energy and improves mood in a *positive* cycle.
- Learning to 're-frame' negative thoughts/beliefs
- Learning problem-solving skills to overcome practical difficulties in life
- Improving negative underlying beliefs and low self-esteem

Making behavioural changes in depression

Changing unhelpful behaviour may be the most effective approach for the limited time-frame of primary care consultations. Teaching patients to challenge and reframe negative thoughts is also important, but can be difficult to use effectively in 10-minute appointments.

Increasing activity levels

One of the key ways to break the vicious cycles of depression is to *increase activity*, particularly if it is pleasurable or increases the patient's sense of accomplishment. Increasing activity has several useful effects:

- Enjoyable activities make life more pleasurable and interesting
- Participating in activities distracts people from continually mulling over negative thoughts that worsen mood
- Success at even small tasks like tidying the house or washing the car, gives patients a sense of achievement and increased control over life
- Increasing exercise may directly alter brain biochemistry and promote positive feelings and improve mood

Depressed patients need to increase activity levels *despite* their negative thoughts or feelings, including lethargy or tiredness. Thoughts such as: "*I can't manage it, I am just too tired*" can be viewed as negative beliefs to be tested out using behavioural experiments, rather than as absolute truth or fact.

Remember that the major difficulty is often *lack of motivation* rather than a physical inability to be more active. For example, a patient who lies sleeping on the couch is still likely to jump up quickly and run away if a man wielding an axe leaped in through the window!

Encourage the patient to behave '*as if*' they are no longer depressed. This involves making positive behavioural changes *despite* feeling tired or lethargic. Choosing small, achievable goals will help build patients' self-confidence and self-esteem.

Initially, the patient may not enjoy activities as much as before being depressed. However, the first step is to restart the activities anyway. Participating in events can still increase patients' sense of achievement. Over time, the increase in activity will help the depression to lift and allow the enjoyment to slowly return.

> ## Case example 12.3: Changing behaviour in depression
>
> George has been depressed for over two years. He feels tired and lethargic and tends to go to bed for a nap when he feels particularly low. George and his GP discuss the CBM and how it applies to depression. When he feels particularly low, he thinks: "*I'm too tired to do anything right now. I might feel better if I rest for a while.*"
>
> George's GP suggests that he could try a behavioural experiment to test out whether this thought is accurate.
>
> They decide to compare two different ways of coping when he feels tired. On one day, he will go to bed and sleep as soon as he feels tired. On the next day, he will try ignoring the tiredness and go for a 10-minute walk or do another activity which might be pleasurable or give some sense of achievement. He will do this on alternate days until he next sees his GP. George agrees to rate his feelings of sadness and lethargy before and after each strategy.
>
> On the next appointment, George reported that he had been surprised to find that resting usually made him feel *worse* rather than better – his mood dropped lower and he usually felt even more tired. However, doing activity had actually lifted his mood on several occasions. He had also achieved several jobs that he had been putting off for some weeks, and felt a sense of positive achievement from this.
>
> After the experiment, George re-framed his original thought "*Resting when I am tired usually makes me feel worse, it is usually better to try to do something more active*" and agreed to continue to gradually increase his activity levels further.

Activity scheduling

Information about a patient's current activity patterns can be gathered using an *activity chart,* which the patient uses to record exactly what they were doing throughout the day (*Figure 12.2*). Monitoring this for a week gives a clear indication of how the patient is spending their time.

If the patient also monitors their mood on the chart, it becomes possible to identify links between the patient's behaviour and their subsequent mood. This strengthens the basis for making changes in behaviour to alleviate depression.

The patient should complete the chart as close as possible to the time of each activity – ideally every few hours – otherwise they may forget what they were doing or exactly how they felt.

Figure 12.2:
Using an activity
chart to monitor
daily activities

Choose a feeling to monitor during the week (e.g. feeling sad, low, empty or anxious)

Feeling to monitor: ....

In each box, write a brief description of the activity you were doing during that hour. Also include a rating of your chosen feeling from 0 to 100 (where 0 is not at all and 100 is the strongest possible feeling) for each activity

Time	Monday	Tuesday	Wednesday	Thursday	Friday	Saturday	Sunday
7–8 a.m.							
8–9 a.m.							
9–10 a.m.							
10–11 a.m.							
11–12 a.m.							
12–1 p.m.							
1–2 p.m.							
2–3 p.m.							
3–4 p.m.							
4–5 p.m.							
5–6 p.m.							
6–7 p.m.							
7–8 p.m.							
8–9 p.m.							
9–10 p.m.							
10–11 p.m.							
11–12 p.m.							

Discussing activity charts with patients

A great deal of useful information can be gathered from completed activity charts, including:

1. Overall activity levels

Identify how active the patient was during the week. Some people may be achieving far more than they realize. Others may be doing very little. Many depressed people will only be doing essential jobs, without any pleasurable activities.

"How active were you during this week? What do you make of this?"

"How much of this activity involved pleasurable or enjoyable things compared to work or chores? How might this affect your mood?"

2. *Variations in negative feelings*

This challenges the belief that 'everything is always terrible':

"Did your mood vary during the week? Can you notice any patterns?"

How does this affect your view that things are 'always bad'?

3. *Links between specific activities and feelings:*

"Which activities seem to improve mood? What other activities which might also be helpful?"

"Which activities made you feel worse? What could you try instead?"

Planning future activities

The next step is to plan ways to gradually increase activity levels. The activities need not be time-consuming or complicated and should be based on what the patient found enjoyable and interesting *before* becoming depressed.

"What was life like before you were depressed?"

"What did you do on a daily basis? What did you enjoy doing?"

It is often also useful to plan activities that may not be fun, but which confer a sense of achievement. It can be very satisfying to complete simple tasks that have been building up for many weeks or months.

To avoid becoming overwhelmed and never getting started, it is often helpful for patients to attempt easier, less onerous jobs first and avoid setting difficult or unrealistic targets. This might involve setting a time limit for the task (*"I will spend 20 minutes on my work project and then stop"*) or by breaking large jobs down into smaller chunks (*"I will just tidy one room today"*).

It can be useful to encourage the patient to produce their own written list of potential activities to try (*Box 12.8*).

Box 12.8: List of potential activities

Enjoyable activities
- Reading a magazine or book for half an hour
- Going for a short walk (e.g. 10 minutes)
- Having a relaxing bath
- Telephoning a friend
- Arranging to meet someone for coffee
- Spending time playing with children
- Other hobbies or interests, including participating in sport

Activities that give a sense of achievement
- Work-related projects or tasks
- Household jobs
- Going shopping
- Organizing finances/paying bills
- Exercise (e.g. walking, swimming, gym)

Next, the patient must plan out which new activities to try:

> *"What activities could you plan for next week, which might help you feel even a little bit better?"*

It is important to define exactly *what* the patient plans to do and *when* they plan to do it. It can be helpful to use an activity chart to plan how to fit in these changes into the following week.

It may also be useful to plan ways to overcome any difficulties that might arise with carrying the activity:

> *"How likely is it that you will actually do this activity?"*
>
> *"What might get in the way or prevent you from doing it?"*
>
> *"How could you overcome these difficulties?"*

Trying the activity

As described above, changes in activity levels should be made *despite* any lethargy, tiredness, low mood or negative thoughts, such as:

> *"It's not worth doing this. I'm not enjoying myself. There's no point. I will never get better."*

The patient should continue to participate and try to concentrate as fully as possible on the activity.

It is helpful if the patient monitors and records their mood before, during and after the activity. This should be recorded as close to the time of the activity as possible, because retrospective recording may result in a negative bias due to a subsequently low mood. Remember that *any* improvement in mood is a worthwhile outcome.

Reviewing what happened

The final stage is to review the impact of the activity. This includes reviewing any difficulties that arose and using a *problem-solving* approach to find ways to overcome them (see Chapter 9).

Successfully increasing activity levels can be viewed as an important achievement and a stepping stone towards making other life changes. For many depressed patients, even simple tasks can be very difficult to accomplish. Patients are likely to undervalue these successes and it is important for the GP to congratulate the patient and remind them not to discount the positives.

Box 12.9:
Summary of
rules for
scheduling
activities

- Use an activity chart to identify patients' activity levels and any current helpful activities that improve mood
- Make a written list of helpful activities to try
- Use the chart to make plans for future increases in activity, including *what, when, where, how long...?*
- Break tasks into small, achievable chunks, e.g. *"I will do 10 minutes of washing up"* rather than *"I must tidy the whole house"*
- Consider how to overcome difficulties that might arise with carrying out the plan in advance
- Carry out activity *despite* low energy or negative thoughts or mood
- Monitor changes in mood associated with carrying out the activity
- After trying the activity review what happened, including using problem-solving techniques to overcome any difficulties that arose
- Always congratulate after *any* success, no matter how small

The importance of physical exercise

Physical exercise has a direct effect on mood to alleviate depression, and is therefore a particularly important activity for the patient to carry out. However, this must also be in realistic and hopefully enjoyable ways.

For example:

- Walks with friends
- Gardening
- Swimming or playing with children in parks
- Fun sports, perhaps with a social element (e.g. team sports)
- Yoga or other gentle exercise classes

Walking is a particularly accessible option, which is cheap and does not necessarily involve a great deal of time. Even a very short walk (5–10 minutes) can be very beneficial to alleviate depressed feelings.

Reminders: Behavioural change in depression

- Increasing activity is a key method of breaking the vicious cycles that maintain depression
- Encourage patients to change activity levels *despite* negative thoughts or feelings such as lethargy by behaving *'as if'* they are not depressed
- Plan changes as small, manageable or 'bite-sized' chunks
- Exercise is particularly effective for increasing energy and improving depressed mood

Case example 12.4: Using an activity chart in depression

Penny has been depressed for nine months. She feels low, tired and has little motivation to carry out her usual tasks. She is very critical of herself for being "useless and lazy" and for "never getting anything done."

Penny's GP explained the CBM of depression to her and how tiredness and low energy are very common symptoms. He suggested that Penny could use an activity chart to check how much she really was doing during each day.

They spent a few minutes during the appointment filling in the chart for that day, to give Penny some practice at using the chart.

Penny was surprised to find that she had achieved more than she had thought during the day. She had got her children up for school, been shopping, cleaned the kitchen and arrived at the GP's surgery on time for her appointment.

Her GP asked how this information fitted with her belief that she was "useless and lazy and never got anything done." Penny replied, "I suppose I do more than I realize."

She agreed to continue filling in the chart for the next week.

Two weeks later, Penny and her GP discussed the findings of her completed activity chart. Penny found that an alternative thought, "I still get all the important jobs done" was more accurate, and helped to lift her mood a little.

When looking at the chart in more depth, they also found that Penny had cut down on many activities which she had previously found enjoyable – she used to swim once a week and sometimes meet a friend for coffee.

The next step was to test out the impact of increasing some more enjoyable activities.

Coping with negative thoughts in depression

There are a variety of ways to cope with negative and unhelpful thoughts in depression. The process of *identifying* and *labelling* negative thoughts helps to strengthen the view that such thoughts are simply *opinions* rather than absolute facts. This helps to promote a more balanced and realistic perspective, which includes both positive and negative factors.

It is important to be aware that the process of identifying and re-living negative thoughts may initially make patients feel worse. However, this may be the only way to challenge such thoughts and make long-term positive changes in mood. Noticing dips in mood caused by negative thinking can strengthen the rationale for using cognitive reframing strategies to improve mood. It is possible to reduce severe distress using techniques such as distraction.

Distraction

Distraction is a simple but effective short-term strategy to reduce the number and impact of negative thoughts. Constantly mulling over negative thoughts makes people feel worse. Instead, concentrating on a practical activity or exercise can distract them from the negative thoughts and breaks this vicious cycle.

Gentle exercise, such as taking a walk or a swim, is a particularly useful form of distraction in depression, as it has the added advantage of concurrently increasing activity and reducing lethargy and tiredness.

Exploring and reframing negative thoughts

As always, the first step involves identifying the negative thoughts that arise during emotionally charged situations, preferably using written CBM charts or thought records. Ask the patient to choose one negative thought to look at in more depth. Then try to identify evidence both for and against it. Finish by asking the patient to try to find an alternative, balanced perspective which includes both positive and negative factors (*Box 12.10*).

Box 12.10:
Questions to explore and reframe negative thoughts

- What is the evidence for this thought? What makes you think that way?
- Is there any evidence against this thought? Is there anything to suggest it might not be entirely accurate?
- Is it logical or realistic? Is it fair? Is there another way to view the situation?
- Is the thought an 'unhelpful thinking style'?
- What are the advantages and disadvantages of thinking this way?
- What advice would you give to someone else in this situation?
- Is there another way to view the situation that takes all of this new evidence into account?

Try to avoid being confrontational or overly challenging during verbal discussions as this may make the patient feel threatened or become defensive. Instead, be genuinely interested and keep an open mind during discussions. Use the principles of *guided discussion* to explore the patients' thoughts, without assuming that you already know the 'answer'.

Case example 12.5: Testing out negative thoughts in depression

Let's return to Roger, a depressed English teacher, from Case example 12.2.

During the next appointment, Roger's GP suggests that he could try testing out one of the thoughts from his CBM chart.

GP Last time we spent some time writing down your thoughts and feelings using the chart. Have you had a chance to take a look at it since we last met? What are your thoughts about what we found?

Roger Yes I did look at it again. It is really interesting to understand more about what happens when I feel depressed. I can see I get stuck in some vicious cycles but I'm not sure how to go forwards.

GP Well, one thing might be to look at the negative thoughts in more detail. Which of these thoughts is the most upsetting or the most important to you?

Roger I'm not sure... perhaps this one: *'I'm a terrible teacher.'*

GP OK, let's write that down. Now, how did you feel when you were thinking that way?

Roger I felt really low and depressed

GP We'll write that down too. Let's look at the thought, 'I'm a terrible teacher.' What evidence do you have that that is true? What makes you think that way?

Roger Well, I'm really behind with lots of my reports and marking at the moment.

GP OK. Is there anything else?

Roger I don't say anything in our departmental meetings.

GP I see. Any other reasons?

Roger I got in trouble with my previous boss for not doing some of my work properly. She said I was too disorganized.

GP Now, is there any evidence that this is not strictly true? Anything that contradicts this thought?

Roger Well, I usually get my work done in the end.

GP Great. Any other reasons?

Roger I do get on well with most of the kids and I enjoy teaching them.

GP That's good. Do you ever get any positive feedback from staff or pupils?

Roger One of the boys from my tutor group came to talk to me about a problem he had. He said he felt he could trust me.

GP Excellent. Anything else?

Roger I had a student teacher sitting in with me earlier in the year and she said she thought my lesson plan was very good.

GP Great. What qualities do you think make a good teacher?

Roger Being a good communicator, caring about the students

GP Do you think you have any of these qualities at all?

Roger Well, I do care about the students.

continued

GP So, let's review what we have been talking about. You had the thought, "I am a terrible teacher." Read through the evidence you have gathered for and against this being true.

I've noticed that there seems to be a lot more evidence *against* the thought than supporting it. What do you make of it all now?

Roger Well, I can see that I do have a lot of qualities that mean I'm not really a terrible teacher.

GP Great, so what might be a more balanced way to look at this?

Roger Perhaps to say that I'm not perfect but I do some things well as a teacher.

Roger's thought record:

Thought to test out: I am a terrible teacher

Feelings associated with this thought: Low, depressed

Evidence *for* the thought	Evidence *against* the thought	Alternative, balanced thought
I'm behind with lots of reports and marking at the moment. I don't say anything in departmental meetings. I got in trouble with my previous boss because I was too disorganized.	I usually get my work done in the end. I get on well with most of the kids and I enjoy teaching them. One of the boys from my tutor group came to talk to me about a problem he had and said he felt he could trust me. A student teacher said she thought my lesson plan was very good. I do care about the students.	I'm not perfect but I do many things well as a teacher.

Reminders: Coping with negative thoughts in depression

■ Discussing negative thoughts may *worsen* mood in the short-term, but is often necessary in order to overcome and change them

■ Distraction offers a useful short-term solution to reduce the volume and impact of negative thoughts

■ Negative thoughts in depression can be challenged and reframed using written thought records

Chapter 13

Low self-esteem

- People with low self-esteem have an overly negative opinion of their own personal value or worth

- It is associated with powerful, negative self-beliefs, such as *"I'm worthless"* or *"I'm stupid,"* which have a major impact on people's lives and relationships with others

- Overcoming low-self esteem involves developing a more balanced, positive view of the self

- People also need to learn to accept themselves as fallible, imperfect human beings

- Assertiveness involves people ensuring that their own needs are taken into consideration by others, *without being aggressive or demanding*

Understanding Low Self-esteem

What is low self-esteem?

Self-esteem reflects the way that people perceive themselves. This includes making judgements about their own personal value or self-worth. When self-esteem is *low*, people tend to view themselves as having little worth or value. They may dislike themselves and are often highly self-critical. Low self-esteem is associated with a range of negative self-beliefs. These exert a major influence on people's lives and relationships with others. Typical beliefs might include:

"I'm worthless."

"I'm unlovable."

"I'm inferior to others."

"I'm weak and stupid."

It is often helpful to differentiate *self-esteem* from *self-confidence*. Self-confidence relates to people's beliefs about their ability to successfully achieve various goals. This may relate to specific competencies such as academic achievements, work success or relationships with others. By contrast, self-esteem reflects the overall opinion that people have of themselves as a person. This is not necessarily related to self-confidence or success. Thus, low self-esteem can occur in people who may outwardly appear to be very successful. In fact, having low self-esteem may drive some people towards continued high achievement in order to internally 'compensate' for their lack of self-worth.

Low self-esteem and other psychological difficulties

Low self-esteem is common. It is associated with a range of other psychological difficulties, including depression, anxiety, eating disorders and social phobia. When depression is present, its treatment should be the first priority, which may sometimes automatically improve low self-esteem. Nevertheless, building self-esteem can also be an important part of the treatment of depression.

Reminders: What is low self-esteem?

- People with low self-esteem usually view themselves as having little worth or value as a person
- They usually hold a range of negative self-beliefs, such as *"I'm worthless"* or *"I'm inferior to others"*
- Low self-esteem is associated with a range of other psychological difficulties and may be a symptom of underlying depression
- People who are highly successful may still suffer from low self-esteem

The CBM of low self-esteem

Thinking styles and cognitive aspects

People with low self-esteem usually experience a wide range of negative thoughts, which are often *self-critical,* or associated with *self-blame* and *self-doubt.*

Several common unhelpful thinking styles are associated with low self-esteem. These often involve a negative or biased view of the self:

- *Ignoring the positive:* Ignore or discount praise, successes or strengths
- *Negative view of the self:* Viewing self negatively, 'self-prejudice.' Focus on mistakes, weaknesses and criticisms
- *Mind-reading:* Negative perception of others' opinions and over-sensitive to criticisms or disapproval from others
- *Self-blame:* taking excessive personal responsibility when things go wrong

Feelings

Low self-esteem is associated with a variety of negative feelings, including:

- Sadness and depression
- Anxiety
- Anger, guilt and shame

Behaviour

People with low self-esteem usually behave '*as if*' their negative self-beliefs are absolute fact. This destructive and self-fulfilling behaviour simply maintains and worsens low self-esteem as a vicious cycle. Such behaviour might include:

- Trying to please others excessively, placing others' needs before their own ("*I am less important than others*")
- Lack of assertiveness or inability to say 'no' ("*I must do what others want, otherwise they will reject me*")
- Underperformance and avoidance of challenges and opportunities ("*There is no point in trying anything – I am too stupid to succeed*")
- Setting themselves up to fail or undermining any chances or success ("*This proves I am completely useless*")
- Perfectionism and over-work ("*I must never make any mistakes otherwise it means I am a failure*")
- Avoiding intimate relationships ("*I am unlovable*") or ending up in abusive relationships ("*I deserve to be treated badly*")
- Avoidance of social situations or contact with others, shyness ("*I am boring and inadequate*")

- Difficulty making decisions (*"I always do the wrong thing"*)
- Poor self-care, such as drinking or smoking too much, using drugs, obesity, not take care with appearance (*"I am not worth taking care of"*)
- Taking excessive care with physical appearance (*"Looking attractive is the only way to be acceptable to others"*)

Physical symptoms

Low self-esteem and the associated lowering of mood may be associated with physical symptoms, such as:

- Physical tension
- Tiredness and lethargy
- Difficulties with sleep
- Changes in appetite and weight

Environment and social factors

Any long-standing environmental or social difficulty can undermine people's self-confidence and result in feelings of incompetence, inadequacy and low self-esteem. This could include relationship problems, financial or economic difficulties, chronic stress, or a long-standing physical or emotional disorder

In these cases, tackling the underlying problem may be the most effective way to solve the problems. However, low self-esteem may also inhibit people's ability to deal with their problems, and it may be helpful to work on this independently in order to support the person in overcoming difficult life problems.

Reminders: The CBM of low self-esteem

- Low self-esteem is associated with negative, self-critical thoughts and over-sensitivity to criticism or disapproval from others
- People with low self-esteem experience a range of negative emotions including sadness, anger, anxiety, guilt and shame
- Behaving 'as if' beliefs about being worthless, stupid or inferior to others are *true* maintains and worsens low self-esteem as a vicious cycle
- Common physical changes include muscle tension, lethargy, tiredness or poor sleep
- Any long-standing social or environmental stressor may contribute to the development of low self-esteem

---

The development of low self-esteem

The negative ideas and beliefs which contribute to low self-esteem are learned from people's life experiences. The development of these beliefs is often an understandable reaction to childhood events or unpleasant, traumatic experiences that occur in adulthood (*Box 13.1*). Most people experience a range of positive and negative events throughout life. In consequence, they develop a complex mix of ideas and beliefs about themselves, which are applied flexibly according to different circumstances. But if people's experiences are generally negative, they are likely to develop predominantly *negative* beliefs about themselves and consequently have lower self-esteem.

Box 13.1:
Negative life experiences associated with low self-esteem

Early or childhood experiences
- History of abuse or neglect (physical, sexual or emotional)
- Being bullied
- Excessive criticism
- Lack of affection or praise
- Rejection by others
- Being different to others
- Unrealistic expectations from parents
- Low self-esteem, stress or emotional distress of parents

Later experiences
- Longstanding stress or hardship
- Abusive relationships
- Being bullied in the workplace
- Experiencing traumatic events (e.g. bereavements, assaults, accidents)
- Loss of status or role (e.g. unemployment, disability)
- Development of psychological or emotional disorders (e.g. depression, panic attacks)

Negative experiences lead to the development of low self-esteem if people view them as a sign of *personal failure or inadequacy*, rather than as simply unfortunate events that could happen to anyone. This is particularly likely for childhood experiences, as children have a tendency to blame themselves for negative events.

Case examples 13.1: The development of low self-esteem

Victor's story

Victor was the son of an engineer. He was a very creative child who loved nothing better than drawing pictures. Victor's father was very scientifically minded. He enjoyed sport and felt constantly disappointed that Victor didn't share this enthusiasm. Victor had tremendous talent as an artist, but throughout his childhood, he was unable to meet his father's expectations in science and sport. He was often told, *"What's the point in that rubbish? You need to achieve something worthwhile."* Victor saw the disappointment in his father's eyes and concluded that he was not

continued

worthwhile himself. His talents and interests were of no use to his father or to anyone else. As an adult, Victor found it difficult to value his talents as an artist and was very self-critical. He believed he was inferior to other people, who he perceived as being more intelligent or educated than himself, and tended to be quiet and withdrawn in their company.

Gemma's story

Gemma was the daughter of a 17-year old single mother with little social support. Gemma's mother loved her daughter but struggled to cope with the demands of a young child. Because of these difficulties, Gemma was fostered several times. She blamed herself for being abandoned by her mother, believing that *"It's my fault she left me. I'm worthless and unlovable."* The constant changing of area and school left Gemma feeling insecure and unstable, and as a result she became moody and sullen. Gemma rarely stayed long with the same family, and blamed herself for this, *"No one wants me around for long – it must mean that I'm a really bad person."* When Gemma was permanently adopted at the age of 11, she was mistrusting of her new family's affection and constantly expected to be rejected again. In adult life, Gemma found it difficult to trust others or to feel secure in loving relationships. She tended to choose partners who let her down and treated her with little care or respect. Even when people did care about Gemma, she found it difficult to believe or trust them.

Bobby's story

Bobby suffered from meningitis as a young child and developed mild deafness as a result, which was not picked up for some time. He was a boisterous child with a lot of energy. He struggled to hear the teachers at school and compensated by channelling his energy into rowdy behaviour and playing around. Because he could not easily follow the lessons, his academic performance dropped compared to his other siblings. His teachers began to label him 'lazy' and 'attention-seeking.' Bobby's parents became frustrated and angry with his behaviour and Bobby was continually in trouble. *"What's the point in trying?"* he thought. *"I'm just stupid."*

Reminders: The development of low self-esteem

- Difficult life experiences may result in the development of negative self-beliefs and low self-esteem
- Negative experiences will cause low self-esteem if people view them as a sign of personal failure or inadequacy
- Experiences in childhood are particularly likely to result in low self-esteem

Overcoming Low Self-esteem

Developing self-esteem involves people stepping back from their long-standing negative self-beliefs and developing an alternative, more balanced perspective. The aim of CBT is for people to learn to view their negative self-beliefs as *opinions* rather than facts, which may be inaccurate, outdated or simply incorrect.

The development of more positive self-esteem includes:

- A more balanced view of the self which includes both positive and negative aspects
- Increased acceptance of the self as imperfect *'warts and all'*
- Increased self-confidence and ability to achieve goals – improved view of own skills, qualities and abilities
- Increased sense of self-worth

Discovering the internal bully

The negative, self-critical thoughts of low self-esteem can be compared to an internal bully. These thoughts can be very powerful and emotionally distressing. It can be useful to encourage the patient to associate this 'voice' with an image – a gremlin, parrot or other imaginary figure sitting on the patient's shoulder and shrieking loud, critical comments into their ear. This can be a fun exercise, which takes a light-hearted approach to understanding the patient's experiences.

By building an image of the criticisms coming from a third person, the patient is able to 'unhook' or disassociate from the thoughts. This encourages the mind to take a more rational view – the thoughts are not immediately accepted as absolute truth or as being entirely accurate.

It can also be useful to consider the *purpose* of this negative critical voice. Just like a nagging parent, the thoughts can be viewed as *trying to help*, by ensuring that the person does not make any mistakes or errors in life. However, this stream of constant criticism is likely to have a negative rather than a helpful effect.

Case example 13.2: Discovering the internal bully in low self-esteem

---

Jessica is a 28-year old woman with mild depression and low self-esteem. She constantly criticizes herself and views herself as unattractive and of little worth. She was bullied at school for being overweight.

In the following discussion, Jessica and her GP discuss a method for Jessica to start to separate herself from her negative thoughts:

GP It seems as if you have some very self-critical thoughts running through your mind...?

continued

Jessica Yes, I am very hard on myself

GP Some people find it helpful to imagine these negative thoughts coming from a grumpy little parrot or gremlin sitting on their shoulder and shouting criticisms and negative things into their ears. Does that image make any sense to you?

Jessica Yes! It is exactly what it's like.

GP What would be the image that comes best to your mind? Sometimes it can be good to make the creature seem a little bit comical or funny.

Jessica I see it as a little wrinkled gremlin.

GP And what kinds of things does this gremlin say?

Jessica Oh... all negative things like: "*Why did you say that? What a stupid thing to do! Everyone will think you are a right idiot.*"

GP And what does it sound like? What kind of voice does it have?

Jessica It is very hoarse and loud.

GP Yes, often, these gremlins have a very loud voice. So loud that it can drown out all the positive and balanced thoughts.

Perhaps we could try to encourage this gremlin to talk a bit more quietly. You could also try to imagine another voice on your *other shoulder,* which is less critical and more supportive.

Jessica That makes sense. But that other voice isn't very loud at the moment – I'm not even sure it is there at all.

GP Well, let's think about this other voice. Perhaps we should look for a more rational and compassionate perspective...

The rational perspective

Being rational involves looking at the *evidence* for a particular thought or belief rather than immediately assuming it is accurate or correct. Each thought is treated as a 'theory' or a 'guess' to be tested against reality.

Rather than being swayed by *emotional* evidence or reasoning ("*It feels as if it must be true*"), being rational involves taking time to carefully consider the situation and avoids jumping to conclusions. This involves weighing up the pros and cons of any particular viewpoint or course of action before making a decision. It may also involve taking a broader or longer-term view of problems.

Box 13.2:
Questions to develop the rational perspective

- How do I know this is true? What is the evidence for and against this viewpoint?
- How else could I view this situation?
- What would I like to achieve in the long-term?
- What is the most important issue to me?
- What would be the most helpful way to approach this situation?

Developing a compassionate mind

A key approach to overcoming low self-esteem is for people to learn to treat themselves with kindness and compassion. This may help to overcome some of the powerful feelings of hurt and distress that may be associated with recurrent, self-critical, bullying thoughts.

Developing the *compassionate mind* encourages people to become their own 'best friend'. This includes patients learning to provide *themselves* with support and reassurance, and to offer themselves the same kind, caring attitude which they often extend to others. Although it is pleasant to receive positive feedback from others, it is important not to depend entirely on others to maintain self-worth. Therefore, as well as learning to get support from others, people also need to learn how to give themselves an internal 'stroke' or 'hug'.

From Theory to Practice...	To illustrate the impact of negative, self-critical thoughts, ask people whether they would talk to others in the same way. Do they use the same torrent of abuse and criticism that frequently runs through their own mind about themselves?
	If the patient would not talk in that way to others, ask *why not?* What impact would it be likely to have on people? How might it affect a child to be continually spoken to in that way?
	Many people with low self-esteem are much kinder, more diplomatic and less judgemental or critical with other people than with themselves. This is useful, as it means that people *already* possess the ability to be supportive and compassionate, and simply need to learn to use same rules and communication styles with themselves as with others.

Being compassionate involves a range of attitudes and qualities:

- Being caring and supportive
- Showing diplomacy and kindness
- Being understanding about difficulties
- Avoiding prejudice (to self and others), being fair and non-judgemental
- Looking for ways to cope with mistakes rather than criticizing and blaming
- Accepting imperfection (in self and others)
- Remembering positive as well as negative experiences
- Not bullying or intimidating others or 'kicking them when they are down'

Box 13.3:
Questions to develop the compassionate mind

- *"What would you say to a close friend or family member if they were in the same situation? What might they say to you?"*
- *"If you wanted to be especially kind to another person in a similar situation, what would you say?"*
- *"How could you look at this situation without criticizing or blaming yourself or others?"*
- *"Are you remembering your own qualities and achievements as well as the negatives or failures?"*
- *"Are you expecting perfection from yourself? Is this fair or realistic?"*

Case example 13.3: Developing the compassionate mind

The following dialogue continues from above, where Jessica and her GP discuss ways to become less self-critical and negative.

GP Could you give me an example of a recent situation where you were self-critical or negative about yourself?

Jessica Yes, last week. I forgot to set the video timer for my boyfriend's favourite show. He said it wasn't a big deal but I just felt so stupid.

GP What kinds of thoughts went through your mind about yourself?

Jessica It was such a simple thing to do but I couldn't even manage that. I felt like such a waste of space. My boyfriend would be better off with someone better than me. I'm not even attractive.

GP I've written down all the things you said to yourself when you forgot to set the video timer: *"I'm stupid," "It was a simple thing to do and I couldn't even manage that," "I'm a waste of space," "My boyfriend would be better off without me," "I'm not attractive"*

Tell me, how does it make you feel to think these things?

Jessica I feel really awful. Just really low and depressed.

GP I think that's completely understandable, given all these critical thoughts that you are having. Now, supposing your best friend had forgotten to set the video timer for her boyfriend, would you say those things to her too? Would you tell her that she was 'stupid' and her 'boyfriend would be better off without her'?

Jessica No. No, I wouldn't say them to anyone else.

GP Why not?

Jessica Because they would really hurt her feelings. It would be a really nasty thing to say to someone.

GP What is your friend's name?

Jessica Helen.

GP What would you say to Helen instead?

Jessica I'd tell her that it's just a small mistake to make. She shouldn't beat herself up about it. Her boyfriend didn't care about it, so why should she?

GP That sounds like really good advice. Supposing Helen keeps saying

continued

that she's stupid and that her boyfriend would be better off without her. If you wanted to be kind and supportive, what would you say to her to help her feel better?

Jessica I would tell her that she was great and that she shouldn't think so badly of herself.

GP How could you convince Helen that she was great?

Jessica I could remind her of all the things she's done well and all the ways she's supported me in the past.

GP That sounds really good. Do you think it might help her to tell her exactly what it is that you like about her?

Jessica Yes, I could say that she is good fun to be with and she's always there when I need her.

GP Excellent. Now, how could you apply all of that discussion to yourself? Is there anything relevant for you in all this?

Jessica Well, I can see that I talk to myself in ways that I would never use with anyone else.

GP And if you wanted to give yourself the same support that you gave to Helen, what could you do?

Jessica I suppose I could tell myself that I am not stupid and try to think up some positive things to say to myself too.

GP It seems like you are already very good at being supportive and caring to other people, like your friend Helen. It might help you to use some of these skills with yourself too. Perhaps you could think about how you might do this over the next couple of weeks.

Jessica It feels very strange but I will definitely think about it.

Reminders: Discovering and overcoming the internal bully

- The negative, self-critical thoughts of low self-esteem are like having an internal *bully*
- Building an image of the criticisms coming from a third person helps patients to disassociate from the negative thoughts and take a more rational view
- The *'rational mind'* treats each negative thought as a 'theory' or a 'guess' which must be tested out against reality rather than taking it at face value
- Developing the *'compassionate mind'* encourages people to offer themselves the same kind, caring, supportive, non-judgemental attitude which they use towards others

Countering negative thoughts and self-criticism

Using written thought records

Written thought records are a powerful way of overcoming low self-esteem by questioning the evidence for and against self-critical thoughts and finding a more balanced alternative viewpoint.

Case example 13.4: Using thought records to overcome self-critical thoughts

Jessica, from the example above, uses a thought record to test out one of her negative, self-critical thoughts:

Thought to test out:

My boyfriend is better off without me.

Evidence *for* negative thought	Evidence *against* the negative thought
I'm not as attractive as many other women. I make stupid mistakes like forgetting to set the video. I'm not as chatty or interesting as other people. I get quite depressed and low sometimes, which difficult for him to be around.	My boyfriend thinks I am attractive – he often says so. He enjoys my company. We have plenty of good conversations. I am a good listener and he appreciates having someone to talk through his problems. I am not always depressed – we do have fun together as well. I am trustworthy and kind and would never deliberately do anything to hurt him.

Alternative/balanced thought to replace the hot thought:

My boyfriend loves me as I am – he doesn't want me to be any different. I have many good qualities and I contribute as much to our relationship as he does.

When a negative thought involves 'mind-reading', it is sometimes helpful for the patient *ask the other person what they really think*. This is particularly helpful with close family members or partners, who may describe many of the patient's positive qualities. However, it can be counterproductive to ask a particularly critical partner or family member, who may reinforce the negative perspective.

From Theory to Practice...

When patients use negative, black-and-white thinking styles, such as *'I'm a complete failure,'* one way to broaden their perspective is to discuss this in terms of a rating scale or 'continuum' (Greenberger & Padesky, 1995a).

Ask the patient what each end of the scale should be, such as 'complete failure' at one end and 'complete success' at the other end:

Failure ———————————————————————— Success

Begin by discussing with the patient what it would mean to be a *complete failure*. Ask them to describe someone who had failed in every possible way. Make sure that the description is as extreme as possible.

Would this person fail to dress themselves in the morning? Would they fail to prepare themselves food? What would their relationships be like with others? Is it realistic for *anyone* to be a complete failure?

Next, ask the patient what a *complete success* would look like. Is it possible to succeed in every single way? How realistic is this? What effect might this have on relationships with others? What might they have to do to ensure success at all costs? Does this make them a nicer or more worthwhile person?

Finish by discussing a more balanced and realistic perspective. The reality is that everyone lies somewhere in between the two extremes. Ask the patient how they could apply this view to their own difficulties.

Identifying personal qualities

It is valuable for patients with low self-esteem to make a written record of any positive achievements and any personal qualities or strengths. This begins to compensate for negative, biased thinking styles that make people view themselves as much worse than they really are.

It may be helpful to begin by encouraging patients to make a list of all their good qualities, along with any *evidence* they have to prove that it is true. People with low self-esteem will often initially find this exercise very difficult. They are used to being extremely self-critical and negative about themselves, and it may make them feel uncomfortable to discuss any positive qualities. They may have a stream of negative thoughts, which discount any positive qualities, such as "*That's nothing special – everyone does that,*" "*I don't do that often enough*" or "*I should have done it better than that.*"

Patients should be encouraged to continue to write down any positive thoughts or qualities and ignore any negative thoughts that arise. Remind them to avoid black-and-white thinking about particular qualities. For example, it is not necessary (or even possible) to be caring or supportive 100% of the time for these qualities to be valuable and important.

The list should include a wide range of qualities. It should include qualities that may not be immediately obvious, but which are nonetheless important and valuable (*Box 13.4*). It is often helpful for the health professional to

Box 13.4: Examples of personal qualities

Kind	Intelligent	Honest
Supportive	Interesting	Reliable
Caring (for others)	Caring (for self)	Punctual
Determined	Successful	Trustworthy
Friendly	Funny	Considerate
Likeable	Smart	Competent
Good listener	Thoughtful	Loving
Helpful	Brave	Enthusiastic
Attractive	Skilled	Taking pride in appearance

spend a few minutes beginning the exercise with patients, and then encouraging them to continue it for homework.

- What good qualities can you notice in yourself? Is there anything you like about yourself, no matter how small it may seem?
- What would someone who cares about you say that your strengths or positive qualities are?
- Think of one or two people who you like or respect. What positive qualities or strengths do you value in them? Do you have any of these qualities to any degree?
- What achievements have you made in your life so far, however small or simple? This might include maintaining friendships, having a job, caring for others, or carrying out hobbies or interests.
- What difficulties or obstacles have you coped with or overcome in your life? Did this involve any qualities such as strength, courage or determination?

Case example 13.5: Identifying positive qualities to boost self-esteem

Jessica is encouraged by her GP to make a list of her positive qualities. She finds the exercise initially difficult but eventually she is able to come up with the following list:

Quality	Evidence that I have this quality
Considerate	"I remembered my friend Helen's birthday and sent her a nice card and present." "When my boyfriend was ill, I did all his shopping and cooked him a nice meal."
Determined	"Even though I was teased at school, I still managed to pass my exams and went on to college." "I keep going to work, even when I feel depressed or low."
Trustworthy	"My boyfriend has given me a key to his house because he trusts me." "Several of my friends have trusted me with personal information about themselves because they say I am a good listener (e.g. Jane, Helen)."
Honest	"I always try to be honest – I have never stolen or done anything illegal."
Caring	"I take good care of my cat." "I often visit my parents to see how they are and try to do things to help them if I can."

continued

Skilled	*"I can cook well, drive and swim."* *"I am learning to use a computer for work – it's not easy but I am improving."*
I am likeable	*"I have several friends who like me; I have known Helen for many years."* *"My boss seems to like me – he is always pleasant and polite."*

Positive diaries

Positive diaries can be used to encourage patients with low self-esteem to look for evidence of personal qualities and strengths. The patient keeps a daily diary or journal, which records examples of achievements, positive qualities or praise received from others.

This process should be continued for several months, to gather a long list of evidence to support a more positive self-view. Having this kind of written information is often useful to call on when the patient is feeling low or discouraged, and has fallen into habitual self-critical or negative thinking patterns.

The diary should include many small examples of positive achievements, rather than waiting for 'major' events. Patients will often discount or ignore things that they view as 'nothing special' or 'unimportant'. However, these small achievements do count and should be included in the diary.

Case example 13.6: Jessica's positive diary

Date	What happened?	What positive quality/qualities does this indicate?
12th March	Tidied up my flat and did my washing Cooked nice dinner for myself	Care for myself Competent
13th March	Invited to lunch with work colleagues Finished my project at work and submitted report to boss	Likeable Reliable, competent
14th March	Went in to work, despite feeling fed up Phoned my sister to see how she is, although I felt tired after a long work day	Determined Thoughtful, caring
15th March	Invited to lunch with work colleagues again My friend, Helen called for a chat and told me about some of her problems at work	Likeable Likeable, trustworthy, supportive, good listener

From Theory to Practice...

It is important for patients to learn to *accept imperfection* – making a mistake or not succeeding in some way is simply a *normal part of human fallibility*. It does not mean that there is something catastrophically wrong with them as a person.

People with low self-esteem frequently focus on one minor problem or mistake and ignore all their positive qualities and achievements.

A visual way of illustrating a more helpful, balanced view may be to draw a diagram, where the person is represented by a large circle filled with dots and crosses:

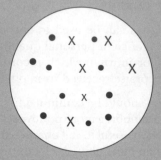

Each dot represents a success that the patient has achieved and each cross represents something that went wrong.

By focusing on one small mistake (illustrated by a small cross) the patient is ignoring all of their other achievements, which are still very much part of the whole.

A more realistic view accepts the presence of both successes and mistakes. *Everyone* makes mistakes sometimes and it is impossible to succeed at everything. Making a mistake or failing in some way does not indicate that the person is a *complete failure*. It simply indicates that the person is normal and human.

Reminders: Overcoming negative thoughts and self-criticism

- Written thought records are a powerful way of overcoming low self-esteem by questioning the evidence for and against self-critical thoughts
- A 'positive diary' involves keeping a written record of personal achievements and qualities
- Self-acceptance involves learning that being imperfect and fallible is a normal human trait

Changing unhelpful behaviour in low self-esteem

Increasing activity levels

Increasing activity is a useful method of improving mood for people who are experiencing low self-esteem associated with depression. It may be helpful to use an activity chart to identify the patient's current activity levels and to plan future changes (see Chapter 12).

The patient should try to reduce self-defeating or unhelpful activities, such as excessive resting or withdrawal from others. It is helpful to take a step-by-step approach to increasing activities which are enjoyable, give the patient a sense of achievement and take into account the needs of the patient well as others.

Behavioural experiments

Behavioural experiments can be used to boost self-esteem by undermining negative self-concepts and reinforcing positive self-beliefs. This process involves devising 'experiments', which test out specific negative thoughts and predictions in practice.

Case example 13.7: Using behavioural experiments to overcome low self-esteem

Example 1:
Negative thought being tested: *I made a mistake at work – this means I am no good at my job*

What could I do to test this thought in practice? (What, where, when…?)	I could ask my boss for feedback on my performance.
What do I predict will happen?	She will say that my performance is very poor.
What problems might arise with this plan?	I might feel too nervous to ask her.
How could these problems be overcome?	I could plan out what I want to say in advance and how I will respond if she is very negative.
What happened when I tried the experiment?	She said that she was happy with my work in general.

What have I learned from this experiment?
Maybe I am more competent than I thought. Making one small mistake may not be a major disaster.

Example 2:
Negative thought being tested: *Jane doesn't like me because she didn't reply to my e-mail*

What could I do to test this thought in practice? (What, where, when…?)	I could phone Jane and ask her if she would like to meet up sometime soon.
What do I predict will happen?	She will ignore my call or make an excuse not to meet up.

continued

What problems might arise with this plan?	She might be out when I call or not answer the phone.
How could these problems be overcome?	If she is out, I can leave a message on her answer-phone.
What happened when I tried the experiment?	She was out when I called, but she rang back the next day and said she was pleased that I had called, and actually invited me out. She said she has been very busy with work recently.

What have I learned from this experiment?
Maybe Jane does like me – she was just busy. I jumped to the worst conclusion about why she hadn't replied to my e-mail.

Reminders: Overcoming unhelpful behaviour in low self-esteem

- A key method of improving low mood is to gradually increase activities which are enjoyable or give the patient an increased sense of satisfaction and achievement
- Behavioural experiments can be used to boost self-esteem by reinforcing more positive self-beliefs and undermining negative thoughts and predictions

Developing assertiveness

Assertiveness means that people ensure that their own needs, feelings or rights are taken into consideration by others, *without* being aggressive, demanding or rude. Learning to become more assertive involves becoming more confident and changing ways of communicating and behaving. It may require a boost in self-esteem for people to really believe that they deserve to be treated with respect and consideration by others.

People often deal with challenging situations by losing their temper, saying nothing at all or just giving in to others' demands. This can leave them feeling frustrated, unhappy and out of control. Both passive and aggressive reactions undermine assertiveness and reduce self-esteem in the long-term:

Behaving passively

When behaving passively, people avoid conflict and always try to please others. They tend to ignore or do not express their needs, and behave as if the needs of others are more important than their own. They rarely express opinions to others, believing they have little or nothing to contribute or that others might ridicule their suggestions.

In the short term, behaving passively may make people feel less anxious or guilty, but by continually sacrificing their own needs, passive behaviour contributes to a continued loss of self-esteem and increased internal feelings of anxiety, depression, anger and frustration.

Behaving aggressively

Aggressive behaviour is often confused with assertiveness, but there are several key differences. People who behave aggressively often express their feelings in a demanding, angry way. This may be based on the assumption that their own needs are more important than other people's. They are prepared to 'win' at the expense of others, by using bullying, unfair tactics and selfish behaviour. This may involve belittling the thoughts, actions or personal qualities of others.

In the short term, aggressive behaviour can help to release tension, make people feel more powerful, and in some cases, ensure they get exactly what they want. However, in the long-term, aggression tends to result in increased feelings of guilt or shame and may decrease self-confidence and self-esteem. Aggression is also likely to damage relationships with other people and may actively *prevent* the person from getting some things, such as support or empathy from others.

Assertive behaviour

Assertive behaviour involves people learning to express their own feelings, rights and needs whilst maintaining respect for other people. This is likely to result in an increase in self-confidence and self-esteem, and an increase in respect from others.

Box 13.6:
Aspects of assertiveness

- The ability to see both sides of a situation and recognize the needs and rights of everyone involved
- Taking responsibility for our own actions
- Asking for what we want, directly and openly, but without undermining others or violating their rights
- Express our own perspective and ensuring our needs are taken into account but not purely focusing on 'winning' or getting our own way, being prepared to negotiate or compromise if necessary
- Recognizing that we have something to contribute to others, irrespective of the opinions of others
- Expressing our feelings in a direct, honest and appropriate way
- Taking responsibility for fulfilling our own needs, rather than constantly depending on others

Reminders: What is assertiveness?

- Assertiveness involves ensuring that our own needs, feelings or rights are taken into consideration by others, *without* being aggressive or demanding
- Both passive and aggressive behaviour undermine assertiveness and reduce self-esteem in the long term
- Assertiveness is associated with self-esteem, as it also involves an awareness of our own worth or value, and our right to care for ourselves, to meet our own needs, to have our own opinions, to say 'no' and to expect others to treat us with respect and consideration

Making assertive statements and requests

When making assertive statements or requests, the first step is for patients to decide what they would like to achieve in a particular situation. This goal should be realistic, fair and balanced. Remember that being assertive does not simply involve people getting their own way, without thought of the consequences for others.

The next stage is for people to express themselves to others, using explanations and requests which are simple and easy to follow. To achieve this, it is essential to keep calm and avoid becoming aggressive or demanding. There are four stages of expressing assertive statements to other people:

1. Describe the problem clearly and objectively
2. Explain how the situation makes you feel
3. Express your needs and what you would like to achieve
4. Explain the consequences of making the change

It is often helpful for patients to plan out ways to increase their assertive behaviour, by rehearsing or writing down what they plan to say.

1. Describe the problem clearly

This should be an objective, factual description of what problem has triggered the discussion, which avoids simply stating opinions, calling names or moralizing.

Don't say	Do say
"You were rude."	*"You interrupted me whilst I was speaking."*
"You were disrespectful."	*"You did not listen to my point of view."*
"I'm treated like a slave in this job!"	*"I've been given more work than it is possible to finish today."*
"The waiter was useless."	*"The waiter was very slow and gave us the wrong bill."*

2. Explain how the situation makes you feel

Use 'I' to describe how the situation affects you *personally*. Remember to take responsibility for the way you feel, rather than blaming others.

Don't say	Do say
"You made me get angry."	*"I felt very angry."*
"You are an idiot."	*"This situation has left me feeling anxious and frustrated."*
"You are overworking me."	*"I feel exhausted and unappreciated."*
"You don't care about me."	*"I feel hurt and let down."*

3. Express your needs and what you would like to achieve

This involves being specific about what you would like to achieve.

Don't say	Do say
"I want you to be more loving."	"I would like you to give me more hugs and for us to go out alone more often."
"I need more support."	"I would like you to take responsibility for some of the housework."
"You never listen."	"I would like you to let me finish my point without being interrupted."
"You need to buck your ideas up."	"I would like you to finish this project by the end of the week."

4. Explain the consequences of making the change

It is helpful to explain what would be the specific *positive* outcome of making the change, for both you and the other person. It is also sometimes necessary to describe the negative consequences of failing to change.

Don't say	Do say
"I need to be taken seriously."	"If you respond to this complaint, I will gain more respect for this company and would continue to work with you in future."
"You need to be a better friend in future."	"Our friendship will be much stronger if I can rely on you to keep my confidences."
"You've got to pay me more attention."	"I would feel happier and more appreciated if you spent some time talking to me about how my day has been."
"You should say what you mean."	"It will help me to do my job more effectively if I have some clearer guidelines about what you would like me to do."

Case example 13.8: Making assertive statements

The following statement includes all four stages of assertiveness:

In a recent report on my work, I was described as lacking commitment and dedication [event]. I feel upset and frustrated by this because I have been working very hard recently on several projects [feeling]. I would like to find out why I was described in this way as I believe I am hard-working and committed and would like to ensure that others are aware of this [need]. This will help motivate me to continue to do my best in this job [consequence].

Learning to say 'no'

Becoming more assertive may involve learning when to say 'no'. The principles of saying 'no' are as follows:

- Be honest and direct about saying 'no', while remaining courteous and polite rather being than blunt or rude
- Communicate the reasons for saying 'no' in simple, concrete terms
- Avoid apologizing or giving complex, elaborate reasons for saying no
- Remember that everyone has the right to say 'no' if they don't want to do something

For people who have great difficulty saying 'no', it may be important to identify any negative thoughts or predictions about the reactions of others if they were to do so. For example, some people may hold unhelpful beliefs or rules, such as "*I must always do what others want, otherwise they will reject me.*"

These beliefs should be identified and then evaluated and re-framed to more helpful perspectives, such as, "*I have the right to look after myself as well as other people*" or "*Others may respect me more if I stand up for my own rights.*"

Reminders: Developing assertive behaviour

- Making assertive requests involves describing the problem objectively, expressing our own feelings and needs, and explaining the consequences of making changes
- It is essential to remain calm in the face of a negative or critical response from others
- Becoming more assertive may involve learning to say 'no'

Dealing with criticism

However carefully people plan out and rehearse their assertive responses, there is no guarantee that others will react favourably to their new behaviour. This is particularly likely if others have become used getting their own way, perhaps because the individual has previously lacked assertiveness and has 'given in' easily or behaved like a 'doormat'.

When faced by unexpected assertive behaviour, people may react by using *manipulative criticism,* which tries to undermine the other person's needs and deflects or ignores their valid arguments or point. There are several methods of coping with reactions such as manipulative criticism:

'Broken record technique'

One of the basic skills of assertiveness involves the person simply repeating over and over again what they want or need, whilst remaining calm and avoiding becoming aggressive. This is a powerful tactic to use when others employ manipulative behaviour, clever arguments or criticism to get their own way. It is also helpful for situations when others say 'no' without a fair or adequate discussion.

Using the broken record technique involves people simply repeating their perspective until the other gives way or agrees to negotiate further.

Case example 13.9: Using the broken record technique to promote assertiveness

Christine is a single parent who relies heavily on her mum, Joyce to help out with her son. Joyce is 59 and has recently started a part-time job as a catering manager in a school kitchen. Joyce is finding the work rewarding but busy and has set aside the evening to plan her menus for the next week.

Christine Would you be able to baby-sit for me tonight? I've been invited to a concert.

Joyce I'm sorry. I can't help tonight as I need the evening to catch up on some paperwork.

Christine Oh, please. It will be such a good show.

Joyce I'm afraid I can't help tonight – I'm catching up on some paperwork.

Christine You could do that any time. I never get out much these days. Surely you don't want me to miss out on this?

Joyce You know that I love to help wherever I can, but I just can't help tonight. I'm too busy with paperwork.

Coping with criticism

It is important for patients with low self-esteem to learn to cope with other people's defensive, critical or abusive reactions to their attempts at being assertive. These responses can be very hurtful, particularly if they contain a small grain of truth. This may trigger powerful feelings of guilt and self-blame in someone with a fragile self-esteem.

In response to criticism, people are often tempted to vigorously defend their position. Unfortunately, this may deflect attention away from their key issues. Instead, they become involved in a major debate or argument about their *own* faults or shortcomings.

A more helpful approach to criticism is to calmly acknowledge that there might be some truth in it. This effectively knocks the wind out of the other person's sails and is a great way to defuse or prevent an argument. Acknowledging the other person's perspective may encourage them to be more flexible and helpful in return. It also helps to maintain focus on the most important issue.

A key factor is for patients to remain calm and take time to think clearly about how to respond to any criticism. It may be appropriate to ask for a short time to think about the comments. When the discussion resumes, the main aim should be to continue to calmly and clearly assert one's perspective. This could include using the broken record technique to emphasize the key message.

Case example 13.10: Coping with criticism

Rebecca is a secretary in a law firm. Her boss works long hours and expects her to keep up with his heavy workload, even though she only works part-time. Rebecca often works late or finishes work at weekends. She is finding the pressure to keep up this workload very tough, as she has a young family which is a high priority for her time. However, she enjoys the work, and does not wish to change job.

Boss Have you finished typing up the case notes that I asked for this morning?

Rebecca I'm afraid not. I have quite a backlog of work from your last case, which I have been finishing today.

Boss Well, I really think you need to learn to prioritize better. I told you this morning that this case is very urgent.

Rebecca You may be right – I hadn't realized that you wanted me to start on this new case before finishing the previous work. But the main problem is that I am being given too much work to manage during my part-time hours.

Boss Your problem is that you are too slow. I need this urgently.

Rebecca I am slow at the moment, because of all the work I have to do, which is impossible to manage during my part-time hours.

Boss Well, I don't know if you are right for this job if you can't cope with the workload.

Rebecca I would be happy to try to improve any areas of my work that you are not happy with. But, I believe it would be impossible for anyone to manage my workload on a part-time basis.

Boss Other people seem to manage – I don't hear any other secretaries in the firm complaining.

Rebecca That may be true – other secretaries may be full-time workers or prepared to work unpaid overtime, which I am unable to do. I enjoy working here and I am keen to do my job well, so I would like to discuss my job description with you and try to make the workload more realistic for my hours, to stop these problems occurring in the future.

Boss Well, you have been very reliable and usually do a pretty good job. We will have to discuss your workload and see what we can sort out.

Reminders: Dealing with criticism

- The broken record technique involves people repeating what they would like or need until the other person gives in or agrees to further negotiation
- People must learn to remain assertive in the face of critical or defensive reactions from others
- This may involve calmly acknowledge that there may be some truth in the criticism, while continuing to repeat the key assertive message

Chapter 14

Health anxiety

- Health anxiety arises from a persistent fear of serious illness

- Patients experience *genuine* physical symptoms, but overestimate the likely severity of the cause

- Anxiety persists despite negative physical examinations, investigations and medical reassurance

- It is important for health professionals to understand how they may inadvertently contribute to the development and maintenance of health anxiety

Understanding Health Anxiety

What is health anxiety?

Health anxiety or hypochondriasis refers to anxiety that arises due to a persistent fear of developing serious illness. Patients without 'real' organic pathology become anxious and preoccupied with their health and misinterpret bodily signs and sensations as evidence of serious illness, despite negative physical examinations, investigations and medical reassurance.

The prevalence of health anxiety in the general population is unknown but it has been estimated that as many as 30–80% of patients who consult a doctor, present with symptoms for which there is no physical basis (Barsky *et al.*, 1990). It is estimated that between 3 and 13% of patients develop hypochondriasis that fits DSM diagnostic criteria (Kellner, 1985).

Cognitive therapy has been shown to be the most effective psychological treatment of both health anxiety and medically unexplained symptoms (Speckens *et al.*, 1995, Warwick *et al.*, 1996, Raine *et al.*, 2002). Although GPs are unlikely to be able to offer 'standard' CBT, it is equally important to understand the key role that health professionals play in the *development* and *maintenance* of health anxiety. This awareness can improve the management of health anxious patients and may limit development of the disorder in some vulnerable individuals.

Thoughts/cognitive factors in health anxiety

Patients with health anxiety are *terrified* about future illness. This usually relates to a variety of misperceptions about health-related issues. Patients with health anxiety tend to:

- Perceive bodily signs and symptoms as more dangerous than they really are
- Believe that specific illnesses are more likely and/or more serious than in reality
- See themselves as unable to prevent or cope with the illness if it did occur

These misperceptions arise owing to a variety of cognitive factors:

1. *Misinterpretation of bodily symptoms*

   Patients with health anxiety tend to interpret bodily sensations negatively and discount benign explanations for their symptoms. This is similar to the catastrophic thinking seen in panic disorder. However, in health anxiety, patients tend to view symptoms as indicating a *longer-term* serious outcome, and consequently develop chronic anxiety responses.

2. *Constant rumination or worry about health*

   Patients with health anxiety spend a lot of time thinking and worrying about health-related issues. These persistent negative thoughts make the patient feel anxious and low and may contribute to other problems, such as poor sleep. Continually thinking about health is likely to maintain patients' awareness of bodily symptoms and worsen anxiety.

3. *Selective attention (ignoring the positive)*

Patients with health anxiety become hyper-aware of information that confirms the idea of having a serious illness and ignore or discount evidence of good health. This frequently occurs during discussions with medical professionals, where patients incorrectly interpret the clinician's words to indicate the possibility of serious illness. This is a common way for misunderstandings to arise in medical communications.

Patients are also highly aware of specific illness-related information in the media. For example, a patient with a fear of cancer may notice all cancer-related stories in magazines, newspapers and on television, whilst ignoring stories about other common problems, such as heart disease. This reinforces their anxiety and fear about cancer, and increases the patient's preoccupation with health-related issues.

Case example 14.1: Understanding health anxiety (I)

Denise is a 35-year old social worker, who is married with three children. In February, she develops an unpleasant viral illness lasting over a fortnight. During this illness she feels feverish, weak and tired with aching muscles.

Denise only expects to be ill for a few days, so she is surprised that the illness lasts so long. A few weeks later she feels much better, but she is still aware that not all the symptoms have completely resolved. She feels weaker and becomes tired more quickly than before. She sometimes feels dizzy and unsteady on her feet, and notices occasional feelings of tingling or pins-and-needles in her hands and feet.

Denise attends her GP on several occasions, who finds nothing wrong. He tries to reassure her that the symptoms are simply due to the after-effects of a nasty virus and will soon go away. But Denise finds that her symptoms do not subside.

Denise becomes increasingly frightened that her symptoms are due to a serious medical condition such as multiple sclerosis. This preoccupies her mind and she begins to feel increasingly anxious. Then she notices a magazine article about a woman with strange symptoms which were ignored by her GP and turned out to be due to a brain tumour. *"Maybe that could happen to me, too,"* she thinks.

Denise starts to think about what might happen if she developed a severe neurological problem. She sees herself in a wheelchair, unable to care for herself and dependent on others. This image is frightening and

continued

upsetting, especially when she imagines being unable to participate in her children's lives.

She tries to block out these horrific thoughts and images, which sometimes helps for a short while. But often, the harder she tries *not* to think about them, the more powerful the images become. Whenever she has a quiet moment, Denise finds herself thinking about becoming ill. But, the more she thinks about illness, the more anxious she feels.

Reminders: Cognitive factors in health anxiety

- Patients with health anxiety misinterpret the meaning of specific symptoms and overestimate the risk of certain illnesses
- They also see themselves as unable to cope if a particular illness did occur
- Constantly thinking and worrying about their health makes patients feel even more anxious
- Health-anxious patients tend to misinterpret medical communications and become hyper-aware of illness-related material in the media

Feelings and emotions

Common feelings associated with health anxiety:

- *Anxiety, fear and panic:* often highly unpleasant and debilitating
- *Low mood and depression:* may be secondary to the chronic anxiety disorder. Depressed people are also more likely to worry about their health.
- *Anger and frustration:* commonly directed at health professionals, who are perceived as ignoring a genuine, severe medical problem

Physical symptoms and biology

Any physical symptom can be associated with health anxiety – it depends on what *meaning* that the patient assigns to the presence of the symptom. This could include assuming that *normal* variations in bodily symptoms and are signs of serious ill-health. Patients may also have symptoms of a genuine physical disorder, such as headache, abdominal pain or tinnitus, but *overestimate* the severity of the likely cause. For example, a patient with abdominal pain may focus on the most frightening explanation of the pain, by fearing that it relates to bowel cancer.

Patients with health anxiety often experience anxiety-related physical symptoms, which are also misinterpreted as further evidence of physical illness. Other factors that alter physiological sensations include the effect of drugs, including caffeine, alcohol or prescribed medication.

Reminders: Physical symptoms and biology in health anxiety

- Any physical symptom can be associated with health anxiety, depending on what *meaning* the patient assigns to the presence of the symptom
- Patients may have symptoms of a genuine physical disorder but *overestimate* the severity of the likely cause
- Anxiety-related physical responses are misinterpreted as further evidence of physical illness

---

The role of behaviour

Common behaviours in health anxiety are designed to check for or protect from physical illness. However, these reactions may actually *maintain* and *worsen* anxiety.

Seeking reassurance

Patients with health anxiety constantly seek reassurance from health professionals, family and friends, hoping to alleviate their anxiety and make sure that there isn't really anything serious wrong. Being reassured by others often helps *temporarily*, but in the long term it simply maintains and worsens anxiety by maintaining a patient's preoccupation with health and encouraging them to monitor and notice symptoms. This results in a longer-term increase in fear and urge to seek further reassurance as a vicious cycle.

Patients with health anxiety often seek reassurance by making frequent visits to multiple GPs requesting repeated investigations or referrals. This can result in frustration and anger on both sides and prevents the patient from building a supportive, trusting relationship with one particular health professional. Different doctors may express inconsistent or contradictory opinions about the cause(s) of symptoms. This leaves the patient feeling confused and mistrustful (*"You can't trust doctors – they all say something different"*). This increases the patient's desire for further referrals and medical opinions, but their increasing lack of faith in medical staff also means that the failure to find a physical cause of symptoms provides little comfort.

Patients with health anxiety often undergo numerous medical investigations, which are often carried out with the aim of reducing their anxiety. However, repeated investigations may *temporarily* reassure the patient, but ultimately tend to *increase* anxiety (*"The doctors must think it's serious, otherwise they wouldn't do so many tests"*). It also reinforces the patient's unhelpful beliefs about the need for medical tests to investigate all symptoms.

Persistent requests for medical intervention may eventually persuade sympathetic doctors to undertake relatively drastic treatments, including surgery or powerful medication. This confirms the patient's fears and may add new iatrogenic symptoms, such as drug-related side effects, which become a new focus for anxiety.

Self focus

Health-anxious patients are very aware of their physical state and may constantly monitor bodily processes such as heart rate, breathing or swallowing. This continual body scanning often results in patients becoming aware of *normal* or *previously unnoticed* variations in body function and concluding that these 'changes' are pathological. This increases their anxiety and generates further anxiety-related physiological changes, which are also interpreted negatively.

Excessive self focus and body-checking will maintain a patient's preoccupation with health and may also cause new symptoms. For example, taking repeated deep breaths to test lung function can cause muscle strain and chest pain. Constantly checking the ability to swallow can result in a dry mouth and consequent increased difficulty with swallowing.

Health-anxious patients may also repeatedly check for lumps, blemishes or other external signs of possible disease. This continual prodding and palpating often causes pain, redness and soft tissue swelling. These signs are also interpreted negatively, and the patient's anxiety increases further still.

Spending time finding out about illness

Some patients with health anxiety spend a great deal of time reading about illness and checking their symptoms against information found from medical books, magazines, TV programmes or searching the internet. Unfortunately, this often increases anxiety, as they discover a whole range of new, potentially serious causes of their symptoms to worry about.

Avoidance

Some health-anxious patients try to reduce anxiety by *avoiding* things that remind them about their health worries. Rather than seeking out health-related information, they avoid reading newspapers or watching TV programmes that may trigger their anxiety and refuse to talk about the illness that they fear. They may avoid visiting hospitals, doctors or other people with ill-health. As in all forms of anxiety, avoidance merely increases health anxiety in the long term, as people never confront their fears or get them into proportion.

Some patients try to suppress or avoid anxiety-provoking thoughts. For some, talking in great detail about every aspect of their symptoms may actually be an attempt to block out the underlying, terrifying catastrophic thoughts of what these symptoms may mean. Thought suppression causes a paradoxical increase in unwanted thoughts, which seem more frightening than ever.

Behaving 'as if' they are ill

Patients with health anxiety often behave 'as if' they are ill. For example, patients with fears about cardiac disease may stop doing exercise, believing that this will protect their heart. Others may use inappropriate medication, corsets or crutches. Taking on an illness role often results in the patient reducing activity levels and may result in tiredness, a loss of fitness and a reduction in enjoyable or meaningful activities in life.

Reminders: The role of behaviour in health anxiety

- Patients repeatedly check their bodies for potential signs of illness and conclude that *normal* or *previously unnoticed* variations in sensations or body function are 'pathological'
- Reassurance-seeking makes patients feel better *temporarily* but causes a longer-term increase in fear and need for further reassurance in a vicious cycle
- 'Doctor-shopping' generates conflicting information and creates doubts about the competency of medical professionals with an increased desire for investigations and referrals
- Unnecessary investigations *increase* a patient's anxiety and reinforce unhelpful beliefs about the need for medical tests to investigate all symptoms
- Behaving 'as if' they are ill reinforces a patient's beliefs that they really are

Case example 14.2: Understanding health anxiety (II)

Denise returns to her GP several times to discuss her fears. As a result, she is referred to a neurologist. She undergoes comprehensive investigations which are normal.

Each time that Denise sees a doctor or undergoes a test that has a negative result, Denise becomes less anxious and worried about her symptoms for a while. But she continues to monitor her body for symptoms, *"Just to be safe"* and after a few days, if she notices any strange sensations, she begins to feel anxious again. *"After all,"* she says to her husband, *"tests and doctors can be wrong. If there is nothing wrong with me, then why do I still feel so bad?"*

In fact, the more she monitors her body, the more symptoms she notices. *"I've got some tingling in my feet,"* she thinks, *"maybe that means I'm having a mini-stroke."*

Denise visits the doctor frequently but feels angry and frustrated because they never seem able to help. She sees a variety of different GPs, who often have slightly conflicting opinions or advice and Denise never knows who to trust. She talks in great detail about every symptom that she experiences, hoping that this will help the doctors to find out for certain what the problem might be. This also helps her to block out the frightening thoughts about what her symptoms might mean.

Because of these continued concerns, Denise spends a lot of time reading medical information and looking on the internet. She discovers a growing list of terrifying-sounding neurological diseases, which might be the cause of her symptoms. She reads these out to her husband, who

continued

usually says, "I'm sure it's nothing that bad. All the tests were fine." This does reassure Denise for a while, but the niggling worries always start to return after a few hours and she starts to feel anxious again.

Denise is particularly concerned that her body feels tired and weak, so she spends a lot of time resting. She keeps a close eye on the power in her legs by constantly tensing and relaxing her muscles, to check that she is still able to move them. However, this seems to make them achy and sore. *"Maybe that's because there is a problem with my muscles,"* she thinks. One day, she tries to hurry to catch a bus and finds that she is out of breath much more quickly than before. *"My health is deteriorating so rapidly,"* she thinks.

Because Denise feels tired, she cuts down on many of her usual activities. She stops walking to work and avoids socializing with work colleagues. She tends to sit down a lot more at home and spends less time playing with her children than before. *"If I feel this tired now,"* she thinks, *"I will almost certainly end up in a wheelchair in the future. My life will be completely shattered."* This thought makes her feel anxious and depressed.

Vicious cycles in health anxiety

The thoughts, feelings, physical symptoms and behaviour of health anxiety usually interact to create vicious cycles of increasing anxiety and fear about health (*Figure 14.1*).

Figure 14.1:
Example of a vicious cycle in a patient with health anxiety

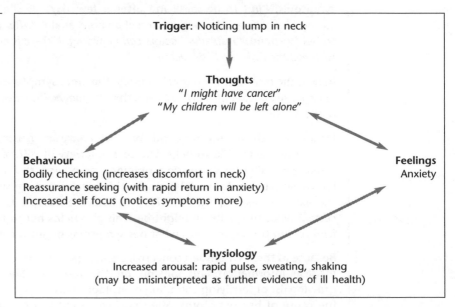

Trigger: Noticing lump in neck

Thoughts
"I might have cancer"
"My children will be left alone"

Behaviour
Bodily checking (increases discomfort in neck)
Reassurance seeking (with rapid return in anxiety)
Increased self focus (notices symptoms more)

Feelings
Anxiety

Physiology
Increased arousal: rapid pulse, sweating, shaking
(may be misinterpreted as further evidence of ill health)

How does health anxiety arise?

Health anxiety develops in vulnerable individuals when a *critical incident* activates specific *unhelpful beliefs about health* developed from past experiences, often during childhood or early life (*Figure 14.2*). A patient's relevant past experiences might include a history of serious illness in themself or family members. This may be associated with the development of beliefs such as, "*People who seem well can often become ill suddenly and die.*"

The interpretations or reactions of key family members to symptoms of illness may also play an important role. Health-anxious patients may have had parents with particular concerns about health ("*Whenever I had symptoms I was taken to the doctor in case it was serious*"). Experiences of unsatisfactory medical treatment ("*The doctors did not find the cancer in my mother until it was too late*") can result in negative beliefs or mistrust in medical professionals.

Figure 14.2:
Development of health anxiety (Warwick & Salkovskis, 1989; Wells, 1997)

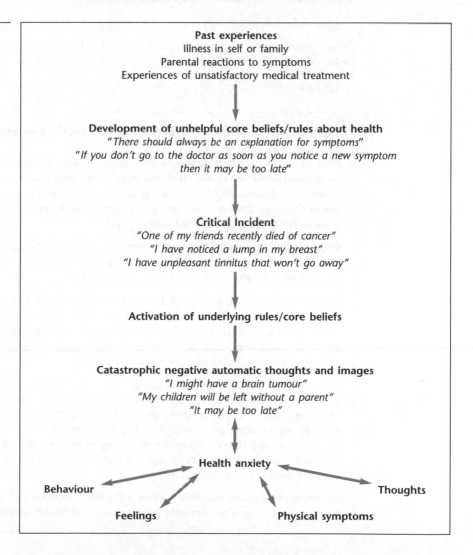

Past experiences
Illness in self or family
Parental reactions to symptoms
Experiences of unsatisfactory medical treatment

Development of unhelpful core beliefs/rules about health
"There should always be an explanation for symptoms"
"If you don't go to the doctor as soon as you notice a new symptom then it may be too late"

Critical Incident
"One of my friends recently died of cancer"
"I have noticed a lump in my breast"
"I have unpleasant tinnitus that won't go away"

Activation of underlying rules/core beliefs

Catastrophic negative automatic thoughts and images
"I might have a brain tumour"
"My children will be left without a parent"
"It may be too late"

Health anxiety

Behaviour   **Thoughts**

Feelings   **Physical symptoms**

A variety of critical incidents can trigger the development of health anxiety, including:

- If the patient develops new or unexpected physical symptoms
- The death of a relative
- Being exposed to illness-related information, such as from the media

Unhelpful beliefs in health anxiety may concern the meaning of physical symptoms or involve the patient viewing themselves as vulnerable to illness, e.g.

"Bodily symptoms mean that there must be something wrong."

"I am weak and particularly vulnerable to illness."

The patient may also have a strong fear of illness or death. This might involve fears about the experience of illness or the loneliness at being separated from loved ones after death, e.g.

"I would not be able to cope with the agonizing pain that always occurs in cancer."

Other fears relate to the potential loss of self-esteem associated with a reduced ability to function normally or work through ill health, e.g.

"If I am unable to work through illness then I am a worthless person."

Case example 14.3: Understanding health anxiety (III)

As a baby, Denise had developed a couple of chest infections and had once been admitted to hospital. Her mother remained anxious about her daughter's health and would keep Denise away from school for very minor illnesses, saying *"Your immune system is weak because you were ill as a baby. We need to take special care of you."*

Denise's mother would take her to the GP immediately any minor signs of illness developed and often said to Denise, *"You can't be too careful. Any symptom might mean something really serious."*

When Denise was 10 years old, her grandmother died. This was a major shock for Denise and her mother. The family felt angry and disappointed with the care that their loved one had received in hospital and blamed medical staff for her death. *"You can't trust doctors – they should have prevented her death. She was fine the day before."*

In later life, Denise remained more aware of her health than other people and worried about any cough, cold or other minor symptom. Then, one of her children developed a chest infection, which was severe enough to require an overnight stay in hospital. Denise found this experience terrifying and it re-awoke many of her childhood fears about ill-health. Although her son recovered completely, Denise found it difficult to manage her own anxiety.

Becoming run down and developing a flu-like illness herself acted as the trigger for Denise's subsequent development of health anxiety.

Overcoming Health Anxiety

Improving relationships with patients

One of the most important goals for GPs should be to build a good relationship with patients with health anxiety. Health-anxious patients genuinely believe that their symptoms indicate a very real, serious, underlying physical disease. This thought is completely terrifying to them. Their understandable reaction is to seek diagnosis, treatment and 'cure' of their problems. When this expected outcome does not take place, despite their continued concerns about ongoing symptoms, patients may begin to feel angry, mistreated and neglected by the medical profession.

GPs may feel frustrated when detailing with a health-anxious patient's repeated attendances, lack of response to medical reassurance and aggressive interpersonal behaviour. But becoming defensive may *worsen* relationships with patients and reinforce the vicious cycle of distrust and anxiety. Instead, try to remember that this behaviour arises from genuine fear. Focus on remaining empathic, open, warm, concerned, respectful and non-judgemental and make a particular effort to develop a collaborative relationship, where patient and GP work together as a team to overcome the patient's difficulties.

It is often valuable to take time to develop an in-depth understanding of health-anxious patients and their underlying fears. This makes it easier to express *genuinely* caring and empathic statements. Because health anxious patients may provoke heartsink responses in health professionals, it may also be important for GPs to carry out some self-reflective work to understand their *own* reactions to such patients (see Chapter 6).

Health anxiety is a complex problem which can be difficult to manage in primary care. Some patients with chronic, long-standing health anxiety are likely to find it very difficult to change their deep-seated beliefs and behaviour patterns. To avoid becoming frustrated and irritated with patients, it is therefore important for GPs to keep realistic expectations about what they are hoping to achieve when working with patients with health anxiety. A more helpful goal may be to aim for 'coping' rather than 'cure.'

Try not to add to problems

The behaviour of health professionals often plays a major role in the development and maintenance of health anxiety. Therefore, it is clearly important that GPs try to avoid contributing to any patient's anxiety. Try to avoid the following unhelpful behaviour:

- Not giving credible explanations for a patient's symptoms, for example by using *negative statements,* such as, *"There is nothing serious wrong with you"*
- Offering repeated reassurance which fails to address the fears underlying patients' anxiety
- Carrying out unnecessary investigations or referrals to specialists

Preventing misunderstandings

It is important to actively prevent the development of misunderstandings about health-related information arising with health-anxious patients. When asking for perceptions of medical communications from these patients, it is not uncommon to hear, "*You told me I have an undetected serious illness*," even though the doctor believes that they said the exact opposite.

Such misunderstandings can be addressed by asking for feedback from patients and by providing written information about their problems. If these difficulties do arise, try not to get into arguments about was or was not said. Instead, acknowledge the patient's perspective and simply reiterate the message that you wish to get across.

> "*I'm glad that we have discussed this as there seems to be a misunderstanding. I may not have been clear in my explanation. What I wanted to get across to you was that…*"

Reminders: Improving relationships with patients

- A key goal is to improve relationships with health-anxious patients, who may feel frightened, angry and neglected by the medical profession
- Health professionals should try to remain empathic, open and non-judgemental
- It may be important for GPs to address their own heartsink reactions to patients with health anxiety
- Patients with chronic health anxiety may have great difficulty in changing long-standing negative beliefs and behaviours
- GPs must try not to worsen health anxiety with inappropriate investigations, unsatisfactory explanations or excessive reassurance

Introducing a cognitive-behavioural approach to health anxiety

Many patients with health anxiety hold a variety of unhelpful health beliefs that cause extreme anxiety about health-related issues, as well as great difficulty in accepting psychological explanations for problems. These patients may find it difficult to accept that psychological or emotional aspects of problems are relevant and may be reluctant to consider addressing these directly.

Rather than trying to *convince* the patient that their problems are *really* psychological in nature, it is more helpful to non-judgementally explore and acknowledge the patient's beliefs. Whatever the cause of the patient's symptoms, it can still be viewed as important to help the patient to learn to adjust and cope better with them.

Reducing a patient's anxiety about health often also involves giving them a *credible and realistic, alternative explanation* for their symptoms. For example, it may be important for the patient to learn that their racing heart is due to harmless anxiety rather than indicating a serious cardiac problem. The aim is not to make the patient's symptoms disappear. Instead, patients can learn that a range of bodily changes and symptoms are normal and do not necessarily indicate serious ill-health.

Improving health anxiety is likely to require a shift in the patient's perspective of what their problem actually is. This may involve learning to accept that a major part of their problem stems from being *worried about* having a serious illness. The impact of these worries may be having a marked negative impact on patients' daily lives.

This change in focus helps to move the discussion towards understanding and evaluating the underlying thoughts and fears that are contributing to the patient's anxiety, rather than continually reviewing and discussing particular symptoms and their possible causes. Nonetheless, it can be difficult to avoid this, and it is common for GPs to find themselves drifting back to repetitive and unhelpful discussions about the likely meaning of particular symptoms.

Case example 14.4: Introducing the CBM approach to health anxiety

Victoria is a 26-year old teacher, whose father died from lung cancer when she was a child. Over the past year, she has become increasingly anxious about her own health, since a close family friend was diagnosed with breast cancer.

She has become increasingly anxious about the headaches that she has been getting over the past six months, despite having been diagnosed with tension-type headaches by a neurologist. She attends the GP surgery regularly, asking for reassurance that the headaches are not serious and hoping for further tests and investigations.

GP Hello Victoria. What brings you to the surgery today?

Victoria It's these headaches – I'm still getting them.

GP I see. What were you hoping that we might do to help you?

Victoria Well, I just think that they might mean something really serious. I'd like to have some more tests to check them out.

GP I've noticed that you have come in several times recently about your headaches, even though you got the 'all clear' from the specialist. You still seem very concerned.

Victoria Well, he might have made a mistake. I don't think it's normal to get headaches so often.

GP You seem really worried.

Victoria Well I am worried. I mean, you read about things all the time – doctors missing things that turn out to be serious.

GP So, worrying about your headaches is having quite an effect on you?

Victoria Yes it is. I feel really stressed about them. If I could just get rid of them, I would be fine.

continued

GP It sounds like there are two problems affecting you at the moment. The first one is having the headaches and trying to work out what is causing them. The second one is coping with all the worry and anxiety that comes from thinking the headaches might be due to something serious.

Victoria I suppose that's true. I am really worried about them.

GP We have spent quite a bit of time looking into the cause of your headaches, but that doesn't seem to be helping you to feel any better.

Victoria Yes, because I just feel that they might mean something really bad. I can't get that thought out of my mind.

GP I wonder if, as well as continuing to treat your headaches, we should spend some time trying to help you feel less anxious and frightened when you have one. This doesn't mean that we stop giving you the medical care that you need. But, it might also be helpful to spend a bit of time understanding why they are causing you so much worry, despite all the negative tests.

Victoria But tests can be wrong! I think I would feel better if I could just be sure that there is nothing bad causing them, or just get rid of them altogether.

GP It is very common to get headaches, so it may not be possible to get rid of them altogether. But, feeling anxious and stressed about having them might actually make them worse.

Victoria I suppose that's true. I know you can get stress headaches. But mine are really bad.

GP Yes, they sound very distressing. Would you be prepared to make an appointment in two weeks time, to discuss this a bit more?

Victoria Yes, I would be glad to come and talk about this. It's all really starting to get me down.

GP Just before you leave, I would like to check that what we have discussed makes sense to you and that I haven't said anything confusing or that makes you feel more anxious.

Victoria Well, you said that I seem very worried about my headaches and that maybe it's because they are due to something serious.

GP I'm glad you brought that up because that wasn't the impression I was hoping to give you. Actually, I don't think the headaches are likely to be due to anything serious. I agree with the neurologist, who thinks they are tension-type headaches. These are unpleasant but not really dangerous. I am concerned that you are so worried about them and I'd like to spend some time helping you to feel a bit less anxious and stressed.

Victoria I see. I'm not sure whether that will help very much but I would be happy to come back and talk about it.

GP Would you be prepared to keep an open mind about what might help? After all, it doesn't seem like what we have tried so far has helped very much either.

continued

> **Victoria** Well, that's true. I am prepared to give anything a go that might help me.
>
> **GP** Perhaps over the next two weeks, you could start to keep an eye out for how these worries are affecting you, discover what impact they are having on your life? I would be very interested to hear when you return.
>
> **Victoria** OK, I will think about all that and come back.

Reminders: Introducing a cognitive-behavioural approach to health anxiety

- The aim of working with health anxiety is to develop a credible, alternative explanation for a patient's symptoms, which does not indicate serious ill-health
- Patients must learn to accept that their a major part of their problem may comprise their *fear* of having a serious illness
- Discussions should involve trying to understand and evaluate the underlying thoughts that are making the patient feel anxious rather than continually reviewing particular symptoms and their possible causes

Working through the stages of the CBM

Discussing physical symptoms

With any patient suffering from health anxiety, it is particularly important to begin by discussing their physical symptoms. This helps to gain the patient's trust and build an effective relationship. It is helpful to spend some time reviewing the patient's physical symptoms while *avoiding* lengthy debates or arguments about the cause or meaning of symptoms.

It is essential to avoid any implication that the symptoms are imagined or 'in the patient's mind'. It is better to acknowledge that the symptoms are *real* and are a source of *major concern and distress*, but they may not be due to serious physical illness.

Discussing thoughts

It is important to identify the patient's most feared medical conditions, as well as identifying their beliefs about what would happen if they did develop the disease, e.g.

> "*When the symptoms are at their peak, what do you think is the worst thing that they might mean?*"

> "*What would be the most worrying aspect about developing this disease?*"

Remember that these thoughts can be distressing and terrifying, so it is crucial to be *cognitively* empathic and sensitive to the patient's distress, e.g.

> "*It must be terrible to be so worried that you have cancer.*"

Discussing feelings

Patients with health anxiety may be unwilling to discuss feelings, sometimes because they are attempting to suppress extreme underlying anxiety. It can be useful to give a rationale for the discussion:

> *"These symptoms seem to be causing you a great deal of anxiety and worry. Is that correct?"*

> *"Perhaps it would be useful to help you reduce these unpleasant feelings, as well as continuing to look at the medical problems."*

It can also be useful to ask the patient directly how they feel emotionally when they experience certain symptoms or think specific negative thoughts:

> *"How do you feel when you think, 'Maybe it's cancer'?"*

It is also important to check for coexisting emotional disorders such as depression or panic disorder.

Discussing behaviour

Ask patients about how they react to their fears, including asking specifically about behaviour such as reassurance-seeking, focusing on the body, behaving 'as if' they are ill and seeking out or avoiding illness-related information. Ask also about the longer-term effects of such behaviours.

> *"How do you behave differently when you feel anxious?"*

> *"What do you do to make yourself feel better?"*

> *"Does it help you to talk to other people about your fears? How long does the effect of this reassurance last for?"*

Environmental factors and triggers to symptoms

Remember to ask about ongoing life stresses and environmental problems, which may be increasing background stress and anxiety levels. It is also useful to ask about specific *triggers* for anxiety, such as reading a newspaper article about heart disease.

It is sometimes useful to ask about previous life experiences, which may have contributed to the development of negative beliefs about health-related issues:

> *"Has anything happened in the past to make you particularly concerned or aware of possible health problems?"*

> *"Was anyone else in your life very concerned about health matters? How did this affect you?"*

Case example 14.5: Working through the CBM in health anxiety

Let's return to the previous example of Victoria, the 26-year old teacher with health anxiety. Two weeks after the previous consultation, Victoria returns to see her GP.

As you read through the following dialogue, try to categorize Victoria's answers into the five areas of the CBM. Can you identify any vicious cycles?

Afterwards, compare your answers to the table below.

GP Hello Victoria. Tell me, what did you think about after our last consultation?

Victoria I've been thinking about what you said in the last consultation and I've noticed that I do spend a lot of time thinking and worrying about my headaches.

GP And do you find that time you spend enjoyable or useful?

Victoria No, it's awful. I feel really bad. But I can't seem to stop worrying.

GP That sounds very difficult for you. Would you be prepared to spend some time discussing things today? I would like to write what you say on a piece of paper, to help us remember what we talked about.

Victoria That would be fine.

GP I would like to start by writing down all the physical symptoms you get that worry you.

Victoria I get really bad headaches.

GP OK, I'll write that down. Do you have any other symptoms that worry you?

Victoria I feel dizzy and a bit sick. Sometimes I feel quite faint. And I get really tired these days.

GP I see [*Writing down patient's words*]. Is there anything else?

Victoria No, I don't think so.

GP Well, we can add in anything else you think of later. Which of these symptoms makes you most worried?

Victoria The headaches.

GP Let's put a circle around that. Can you think of a recent time that you had a headache that worried you?

Victoria Yes, last week, after work.

GP Right. Tell me what went through your mind when you noticed the headache?

Victoria I just felt sure that it must be something serious. The pain is just so bad.

GP And how did that make you feel emotionally?

Victoria I felt really anxious and tense.

GP What was making you feel so anxious? What might 'something serious' be?

continued

Victoria I suppose I have a worry that it could be a brain tumour.

GP That must be a very scary thought.

Victoria It is – it's terrifying.

GP What makes you think it might be a brain tumour?

Victoria Because the pain is very severe, and I've had these problems for a long time without getting any better. I read a medical book and it said that headaches can be caused by all kinds of serious things.

GP I see. That makes sense. Could you tell me what is the most terrifying part about having a brain tumour? What do you imagine would happen to you?

Victoria [*Looks tearful*] I remember my dad when he died from lung cancer. He was in so much pain. I just don't think I could cope with it.

GP That must have been a very difficult experience for your whole family.

Victoria Oh yes, it was really tough for all of us to see him so ill, in so much pain. But there was nothing we could do to help.

GP That sounds really tough. Do you think that experience has any effect on how worried you tend to get when you have symptoms like a headache?

Victoria I suppose it might. I know I always think the worst whenever I get ill – I start worrying it could be something bad, like my dad. He had a cough for ages that the doctors just ignored.

GP How do you react when you get a headache? What do you do differently?

Victoria I usually take some tablets and go to bed for the rest of the evening.

GP You mentioned that you have looked in a medical book about headaches. Is that something you do often?

Victoria Well, I look on the internet and in books to try to find other ways to help me or to work out what the problem is.

GP And what have you found out?

Victoria Well, there seem to be so many different things that it could be. Some of them sound really bad, like swelling on the brain or an aneurism.

GP How does it make you feel emotionally to think about all these things that could be causing your headaches?

Victoria I feel really worried. Sometimes I feel really terrified [*Begins to look very anxious*]. Do you think they are caused by something like that?

GP It must be really frightening to believe that your headaches may be caused by something so serious. Can you remember what we talked about at the end of the last appointment, about what I think is causing your headaches?

Victoria No, I'm not sure.

GP Try to think back. We talked about the most likely cause of your headaches.

continued

Victoria Oh, yes. You said something about being tension headaches.

GP Yes, well done for remembering. I noticed something really interesting just then. When you started to think about the most severe causes of your headaches, you became very anxious.

Victoria Yes, that's true. I hadn't really realized before.

GP What do you make of that?

Victoria I suppose thinking about all these scary diseases makes me feel very anxious.

GP That could be a really useful thing to have found out, if you are hoping to feel less anxious. I've also noticed that you seem to feel less worried if I reassure you that the problem isn't serious. Is that correct?

Victoria Yes, I do feel better.

GP And do you ever ask anyone else to reassure that things are OK?

Victoria Well, I often phone up my mum. She always says the headaches are nothing to worry about.

GP So you tend to feel better if people reassure you?

Victoria Yes, I suppose it reminds me that it probably isn't anything too serious after all.

GP And how long do you feel better for? Is there anything that I could say that would stop you *ever* becoming anxious again?

Victoria Well, it lasts for a few days or maybe even less. As soon as I get another headache I feel anxious again.

GP So reassurance doesn't help much in the long-term. That's interesting too. It can sometimes be more helpful to learn how to *reassure ourselves* rather than always turning to others.

Victoria That makes sense, but I don't know how to do that. When I feel worried, I just feel that the only thing that might help is to talk to someone else.

GP OK, Victoria. We are nearly out of time today, so I would like to summarize everything we have said and then ask what you think about it all...

Victoria's CBM chart:

Situation: Developing a headache after work on Thursday evening

Thoughts	Feelings
"It must be something serious – the pain is so bad."	Anxious
"It could be a brain tumour."	Tense
"I couldn't cope with the terrible pain that my dad had."	Worried
"When I feel worried, the only thing that might help is to talk to someone else."	Terrified
Unhelpful thinking style: Automatically thinking the worst about the cause of all symptoms	

continued

Behaviour	Physical symptoms/ biology
Take some tablets and go to bed for the rest of the evening	Headaches
Look on the internet and in medical books – discover lots of serious possible causes of headaches	Dizziness
Ask other people (GP, mum) for reassurance	Feel sick
	Feel faint

Environmental factors/triggers
Dad died from lung cancer in a lot of pain
The doctors ignored Dad's cough and it turned out to be something very serious

Reminders: Working through the stages of the CBM

- Begin by reviewing the patient's physical symptoms, but avoid lengthy debates or arguments about the cause or meaning of symptoms
- Identify the specific thoughts and feelings that arise in the patient when they experience specific physical symptoms
- Try to discover a patient's worst fears about what symptoms might mean, as well as what they believe would happen if they did develop the disease that they fear
- Look for environmental factors, both past and present, which may make patients vulnerable to anxiety about health issues

Looking for alternative explanations for symptoms

Using a pie chart to generate alternative ideas for symptoms

A pie chart can be a powerful, visual tool, which encourages the patient to keep in mind the most common and likely causes of particular symptoms. Use the principles of guided discovery to encourage patients to think up a range of possible causes and to draw their own conclusions from the exercise.

Case example 14.6: Using pie-charts to look for alternative explanations for symptoms

Let's return to the example of Victoria, the young woman with headaches and health anxiety.

Her GP encourages her to generate a list of common causes for headaches:

continued

- Stress and tension
- Migraine
- Eye strain/bright light
- Loud noise
- Bang on the head
- Blocked sinuses
- Meningitis
- Aneurism
- 'Swelling of the brain'
- Brain tumour

Next, Victoria's GP draws a large circle and asks Victoria to divide up the 'pie' into slices. Each slice represents how common the different causes are and how likely to have caused headaches in a woman of her age. She leaves her most feared cause (a brain tumour) until *last* to put on the chart.

She draws the following pie-chart:

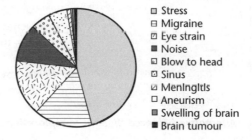

□ Stress
⊟ Migraine
▨ Eye strain
■ Noise
▨ Blow to head
▨ Sinus
▨ Meningitis
□ Aneurism
▨ Swelling of brain
■ Brain tumour

After this exercise, Victoria's GP asks her, *"What do you make of this chart?"* Victoria replies that it is helpful to think about all the possible causes of her illness rather than focusing on the one or two, most serious possibilities.

Note for GPs:
There is no need for the chart to be divided with absolute precision or accuracy. The sections need only be approximate. But if the patient is overestimating the likelihood of a particular cause, it may be helpful to discuss this openly with them.

Looking for evidence for and against specific, feared diagnoses

It can be helpful to use written thought records to look for evidence for and against particular negative thoughts or feared diagnoses.

> ### Case example 14.7: Using thought records to test out unhelpful thoughts in health anxiety
>
> Victoria used the following thought record to challenge her fears of having a brain tumour:
>
> **Thought to test out:** *My headaches are due to a brain tumour.*
>
> | Evidence *for* having a brain tumour | Evidence *against* having a brain tumour |
> | --- | --- |
> | The headaches I get are very severe.
I have had them for a long time.
Doctors do make mistakes and sometimes miss serious illnesses. | Brain tumours are very rare – there are many other causes of headaches and most are not serious.
I have had lots of tests, including a brain scan. These were all normal.
The headache gets better if I lie down and rest – brain tumours would not get better so easily.
My headaches are worse when I am stressed or anxious – this does not fit with having a brain tumour.
The doctor says that I do not have any other signs that would indicate a brain tumour. |
>
> *Alternative/balanced thought to replace the hot thought:*
>
> My headaches are more likely to be due to tension and stress. Worrying about my headaches makes them worse and makes me feel very anxious.

Other methods of coping with anxiety and worry

Useful strategies to deal with anxiety-provoking thoughts include:

- Using distraction to focus the mind on other things
- Using a 'then what..?' approach to identify ways to cope with fears. For example, discussing how to cope if they did develop a feared disorder.
- Have a designated 'worry time' of perhaps half an hour per day – the patient can tell themselves that there is no need to worry *all* the time, because they can do it later

Learning to cope with uncertainty about health

It is impossible to completely eliminate the risk of developing *any* disease, no matter how rare it may be. But the chance of developing a serious illness is very low, particularly if medical investigations or tests are normal. However, health-anxious patients often state that they would like to be *certain* that nothing serious is wrong.

It can be helpful to remind patients that every person must cope with uncertainty and risk every single day of their lives. Every time we cross the road, we risk being hit by a car. As we leave our home, we run the risk of being struck and killed by a stray meteorite. *Nothing* is completely safe. It is important to take every reasonable precaution against these possibilities, but it is impossible to eliminate risk altogether.

Spending all our time worrying about developing an illness does not make it any less likely to occur! Always focusing on the worst case scenario simply increases the levels of stress and anxiety in life. A more helpful approach is to assess how great the risk *really* is and then get on with the rest of life.

Reminders: Looking for alternative explanations for symptoms

■ Pie-charts are a visual method of encouraging the patient to consider less serious or devastating causes for symptoms
■ Written thought records can be used to seek evidence for and against the most feared causes of particular symptoms or other unhelpful thoughts
■ Distraction may help manage high levels of anxiety
■ It may be useful to plan how patients could cope if they really did develop a feared disorder

Overcoming unhelpful behaviour in health anxiety

Promoting behavioural change is one of the most powerful strategies for dealing with health anxiety. This includes looking for the *pros* and *cons* of existing behaviour patterns and identifying new, more helpful alternatives.

It is often helpful to use behavioural experiments to help patients discover the unhelpful effects of behaviour such as reassurance seeking and body checking.

From Theory to Practice...

Investigating the effect of reassurance

Ask patients with health anxiety to observe and record the effects of other people's reassurance on their anxiety.

Does it alleviate their anxiety? How long does this last for?

Does having reassurance reduce any anxiety-related symptoms? Would a serious diagnosis be likely to go away simply with reassurance?

Looking at the effect of monitoring and body-checking behaviour

Ask patients to notice what happens when they focus internally on symptoms or their body state. How does this alter their thoughts or anxiety levels?

Encourage the patient to discover the effect of body-checking behaviour. What is the impact of continually poking and prodding the skin or of continually taking forced, deep breaths? How might this contribute to their anxiety problems?

Minimizing reassurance-seeking

Patients should be encouraged to reduce seeking reassurance from others. This includes trying to stop asking doctors, family and friends about their health. It may be helpful to involve a patient's family, by asking them not to offer reassurance or to change the subject if the patient begins talking about their health. To avoid conflict, these strategies should be agreed in advance.

Instead of seeking reassurance, the patient could try a range of other activities, such as going for a walk, doing a household chore or a hobby, and monitor the impact this has on their mood. They could also try to reassure themselves using pre-planned, written information. This could include re-reading previously constructed pie-charts, thought records or written strategies for how to respond to anxiety-provoking situations.

It can be useful for the patient to keep a diary of how often they ask for reassurance. This helps to monitor how frequent this behaviour is and whether they are successfully managing to reduce how often they ask for reassurance.

It is also useful to reduce reassurance from health professionals. This should include an explicit discussion and agreement *in advance* of how the GP will subsequently respond to requests for reassurance. For example:

> *"It sounds like you are asking me for reassurance. We discussed this last week and discovered that it doesn't really help you in the long-term. If you think back to conversations we have had in the past, can you remember any helpful information that might help you reassure yourself?"*

Reducing monitoring and body checking

Health-anxious patients often check their bodies for potential problems many times each day. It is helpful to ask patients to record how often they check a particular aspect of their physical health. This could be recorded in a journal or using a daily chart, similar to the activity charts used in depression (Chapter 12). It is often useful to monitor both short- and long-term changes in anxiety levels associated with body checking.

The next step is to agree how much body checking is *helpful* and to plan how often the patient will check in future. For example, if the patient fears cancer, then checking once a month may be more realistic and helpful than checking several times an hour.

It is often difficult to stop body checking, which may have become an ingrained *habit*. Techniques such as distraction or using thought records to find alternatives for negative thoughts are sometimes useful. Patients can also remind themselves that body checking is increasing their anxiety in the long term.

Stop behaving 'as if' they are ill

It is particularly important for patients to gradually resume their normal daily activities. Just as in depression, this is likely to boost mood, increase the level of enjoyment in life, give patients an increased sense of satisfaction and take their minds off negative thoughts and worries.

To identify useful behavioural changes, ask the patient:

> *"What was life like before you developed these symptoms?"*
>
> *"If you woke up tomorrow and your problems had magically all been solved, what would be different?"*

This can help to identify a list of activities, which can be gradually increased over time.

Reducing time spent finding out about illness

Encourage health-anxious patients to reduce excessive time spent thinking about illness by reducing how often they read about it, watch medical programmes or make health-related internet searches.

Reducing avoidance of illness-related topics

For patients that avoid thinking or talking about health-related subjects, it can be helpful to face their fears. It is often useful to identify and actively challenge their underlying anxiety-provoking thoughts, using a written thought record. Patients could also be encouraged to overcome avoidance using graded exposure to a hierarchy of increasingly anxiety-provoking situations.

Reminders: Key behavioural changes in health anxiety

- Reduce reassurance-seeking
- Reduce body checking
- Stop behaving 'as if' they are ill
- Reduce time spent finding out about illness
- Reduce avoidance of health-related topics

Chapter 15

Psychological aspects of chronic physical disease

- The CBM can be used to identify psychological, emotional and behavioural aspects of chronic physical disease

- Psychological disorders such as depression and anxiety may be more common in patients with physical disorders but are under-diagnosed and under-treated

- Increasing positive activities and improving mood can often reduce the intensity or emotional distress associated with unpleasant symptoms

- Understanding negative beliefs about health and illness may help to improve management of certain conditions, including compliance with treatment

- The aim is to enhance coping with unpleasant physical symptoms, such as chronic pain, rather than trying to eliminate them entirely or 'cure' the patient

The psychological impact of chronic disease

Chronic medical conditions have become increasingly prevalent and comprise a large part of the primary care workload. People are living longer and medical conditions that used to result in a high mortality are managed more effectively. As a result, a large number of the population must learn to live with chronic disease for a significant part of their lives. But this conflicts with increasingly high public expectations of the medical profession. Many people now believe that medical advances mean that virtually all medical problems can or should be 'cured'. This makes it more difficult to accept or cope with long-standing chronic illness or disability.

Developing chronic illness or disability often has a major psychological impact and is likely to require major changes in people's attitudes and lives. Patients need to learn to cope with their disease and its associated symptoms. This includes adjusting to changes in bodily functioning, which may vary from day to day. Patients must also make psychosocial adjustments, including finding ways to maintain independence and previous roles. People with chronic disease must also deal with uncertainty as to the possible future or prognosis of the illness, which often involves a probable long-term decline in health status.

Patients also have to learn to understand and manage their medical condition. Learning to cope with the requirements of monitoring and treating a disease is often more challenging than dealing with the illness itself. Some treatments produce unpleasant side effects or require unwelcome life changes.

Overlap between physical and emotional disease

Emotional disorders are common in patients with physical disease and around 20–25% of patients with chronic medical problems experience clinically significant psychological symptoms such as depression or anxiety (Craig & Boardman, 1997). However, health professionals often focus predominantly on the *physical* rather than the *emotional* health of patients with chronic disease, and depression is more likely to be *missed* or overlooked in these patients.

Patients with chronic disease may also have coexisting psychological problems, which may be worsened by the additional difficulty of experiencing chronic disease. Other patients develop somatization disorders, where underlying psychological distress is expressed as physical, somatic symptoms.

The role of health beliefs in chronic disease

People's beliefs about the diagnosis, symptoms, severity, duration and cause of their illness, as well as their views about the value or role of medical or other treatments, will affect how they make sense of or give meaning to their illness. These beliefs influence individual coping strategies, behavioural reactions to illness, compliance with treatment and the emotional impact of health problems. It may also affect the overall outcome for the patient in terms of both physical and mental well-being.

Certain beliefs about illness may predispose the patient to becoming depressed, anxious or angry in the face of real or potential illness. These may involve a variety of areas:

Loss of identity or role:	*"Being unable to work means I have nothing to offer."* *"Being ill is a sign of weakness."*
Judgement of others:	*"Others think less of me for being ill."*
Views about treatments:	*"Medications are dangerous and should be avoided."*
Negative predictions of future:	*"Nothing can help me."*
Perception of own health status:	*"My body is weak and needs as much help as possible."*
Beliefs about meaning of symptoms:	*"I can only feel better if I am completely free from all symptoms."* *"If I have a new symptom it means my illness has progressed."*

When people hold these kinds of negative or unhelpful beliefs, they may adopt a variety of unhelpful coping strategies and safety behaviours in response to physical illness. This might include lack of compliance with treatment regimes, excessive reassurance-seeking or social withdrawal from others. These behavioural patterns can lead to worsening low mood, increased anxiety and low self-esteem.

Spending time identifying and addressing a patient's unhelpful health beliefs can be an effective method of improving both physical health and emotional well-being. It may be possible to identify more helpful ways for patients to view themselves and their illness. This process may encourage patients to adopt more positive coping strategies and can reduce emotional distress. For example:

"I am a worthwhile, valuable person, despite no longer working."

"It is normal and human to become ill."

"Medications may sometimes be necessary to help my body."

"Others will still respect and care for me if I become unwell."

"The worst may not happen."

"I can cope with the problems that I am facing."

Reminders: The psychological impact of chronic disease

- Chronic, incurable medical conditions are increasingly common
- Learning to cope with chronic disease is likely to require major changes in people's attitudes and lives
- Emotional disorders such as depression and anxiety are common amongst people with chronic physical disease but are more likely to be overlooked by health care professionals
- People with negative or unhelpful health beliefs may be vulnerable to developing psychological difficulties or emotional distress if they become chronically unwell

Using the CBM with physical illness and disability

Aims of using the approach

The CBM is a very effective method of understanding the psychological aspects of adjusting to and coping with chronic physical disease. It provides a generic approach that is useful for understanding the difficulties associated with a variety of medical problems.

The goal for managing chronic disease is to promote independence and enjoyable living, *despite* the presence of chronic disease. It does not promote an unrealistically positive view, but encourages patients to take a balanced perspective of themselves and their lives. This may involve learning to *accept* alterations in body function, appearance and lifestyle, without associating these changes with a loss of personal worth or value.

Identifying and changing any unhelpful behaviour patterns is a key strategy for promoting positive change. For example, patients may behave 'as if' they are more unwell or disabled than is really the case, which limits activity and can worsen mood.

Introducing the CBM to patients with physical disorders

The CBM can be introduced to patients as a way of providing an overview or map of the problems that exist in different areas of their lives. This includes difficulties related to physical ill-health, as well as other, unrelated problems. For example, the model could be introduced to a patient with chronic pain in the following way:

> "*I have seen you several times for this pain. It seems very distressing for you. I wonder if it would be helpful to look at the specific ways that it affects your life, as pain can affect people in different ways.*
>
> *This means talking about all the things going on in your life at the moment. Of course, it doesn't mean that I think the pain isn't really distressing or that it is all 'in your mind.' We will continue to look after your physical health, just as before.*
>
> *The process may help us to think up some new ways to help you, or it may be that we just understand what is going on a bit a better.*"

Case example 15.1: Using the CBM in diabetes

Donald is a 56-year old, overweight decorator who was diagnosed with type II diabetes last year during a routine health check. His blood sugar readings indicate that his diabetes is poorly controlled but he does not appear interested in his illness. Donald's GP suspects that he is not taking his medication regularly, as he rarely asks for a repeat prescription. But whenever the practice nurse tries to educate him about diabetes and encourage him to take his medication, he gets irritated and aggressive, saying that he has "heard it all before."

Simply lecturing Donald unsuccessfully has been causing frustration for both GP and patient, so Donald's GP decides to use the CBM to gain a greater understanding of Donald's reluctance to discuss diabetes or take his medication.

Thoughts
"Having diabetes means that I am 'ill' and my body is weak and out of control."
"If I think too much about diabetes it will take over my life – better to ignore it."
"It is dangerous to take medications – my uncle got an ulcer from his tablets last year."

Behaviour
'Forgets' tablets – so diabetes gets out of control
Avoids thinking about health
Fails to exercise or lose weight

Feelings
Fed up/low
Anxious

Physical symptoms
Tired and lethargic

Environment
Donald doesn't really enjoy his job – *"It pays the bills"*
His friends are mainly in his local pub – most drink quite heavily
His wife is also overweight and tends to cook rich and fatty food

Potential outcomes from using the model:
By understanding Donald better, the GP feels less frustrated and is able to express genuine empathy for the patient's difficulties. This helps improve their relationship, and encourages Donald to attend the diabetic clinic more regularly.

Donald and his GP are able to discuss the evidence for and against his negative thoughts and beliefs about diabetes. They may be able to develop some alternative, more helpful ways to view diabetes, such as:

continued

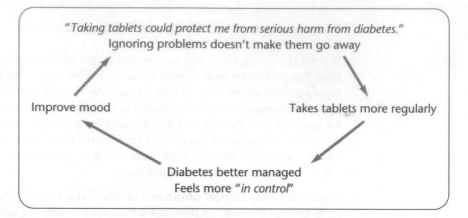

"*Taking tablets could protect me from serious harm from diabetes.*"
Ignoring problems doesn't make them go away

Improve mood

Takes tablets more regularly

Diabetes better managed
Feels more "*in control*"

Case example 15.2: Using the CBM in asthma

Benjamin is a 23-year old history student who suffers from asthma. He regularly attends the asthma clinic, which is run by the practice nurse. She has stepped up his treatment following the asthma guidelines. She is concerned that he remains very anxious about his condition and asks for frequent repeat prescriptions of his salbutamol inhaler, despite his regular, preventative inhalers and good objective measures of his asthma, such as peak flow. He also regularly requests 'emergency' consultations to review his asthma and often seems anxious when he attends the surgery.

Benjamin's GP decides to review the young man's concerns about his asthma using the CBM and discovers that he is under a lot of pressure in his final year at university:

Triggers for feeling anxious/worsening asthma: Having a deadline for an essay

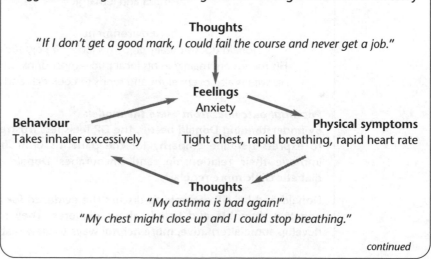

Thoughts
"*If I don't get a good mark, I could fail the course and never get a job.*"

Feelings
Anxiety

Behaviour
Takes inhaler excessively

Physical symptoms
Tight chest, rapid breathing, rapid heart rate

Thoughts
"*My asthma is bad again!*"
"*My chest might close up and I could stop breathing.*"

continued

> **Environment/social factors**
> Final year of history degree
> Uncertain what career choice he is hoping for
> Parental pressure to succeed in life (his brother is a high-earning
> City banker)
>
> This discussion gives both GP and patient more insight into Andrew's behaviour patterns. It helps to educate Andrew about the relationship between asthma and anxiety symptoms. Andrew realizes that learning to manage his anxiety is likely to help his physical symptoms and improve his asthma control, as well as cut down the use of his inhaler. This enables him to find ways to break this vicious cycle, whilst maintaining good control of his asthma.

Reminders: Using the CBM with physical illness and disability

- The aim is to promote the patient's independence and enjoyment of life, despite the presence of chronic disease
- Patients may benefit from taking a more balanced perspective, which does not associate illness with a lack of self-worth or personal value
- The CBM can also be useful to understand conditions with elements of both physical and psychological problems

Depression and chronic physical disease

Depression is common amongst patients with chronic physical disease (Peveler, Carson & Rodin, 2002), but its diagnosis is not always straightforward in this group. Biological features of depression such as fatigue and lethargy may be confused with physical symptoms associated with the patient's medical condition. Patients may also be unwilling to report symptoms of depression. Some drug treatments may also *cause* depression as a side effect, such as corticosteroids, anti-parkinsonian drugs, some antihypertensive medication (methydopa, clonidine), and chemotherapy agents (vincristine, vinblastine).

Depression in patients with chronic physical disease can be effectively treated, and should be appropriately assessed and managed, just as in any other depressed patient (Chapter 12). This could include the use of antidepressant medication or psychological approaches/therapy.

Strategies for overcoming depression

- Cognitive strategies: identify and reframe negative or unhelpful thoughts
- Encourage patients to share concerns and seek support from friends and family
- Building self-esteem: use positive diaries or lists of personal qualities to re-build self-esteem, despite the presence of illness

- Activity scheduling: increase enjoyable activities, as well as those which give the patient a sense of independence and achievement
- Increase social interaction
- Exercise

Case example 15.3: Depression and chronic disease

Diane is a 45-year old woman with multiple sclerosis. Her physical strength and mobility has gradually reduced over the past five years and she is now largely confined to a wheelchair. She is married with two children and feels increasingly low about her loss of independence and difficulty carrying out her normal tasks of daily living. She is no longer able to play physical games with her children, or to lift her youngest son, Ivan, aged 4.

Thoughts	*"I'm a terrible mum – I can't even play with the children any more."* *"I've failed my family."* *"Things are only going to get worse in the future."*
Feelings	Guilt, depression
Behaviour	Reduced interaction with her children (she feels guilty and reminded of her inability when she does so). This reinforces her belief about being a 'bad' parent. Frequently mentions her perceived 'failure' to her husband, Barry. This type of conversation makes him feel anxious and low, so he usually responds by changing the subject. Diane views this reaction as 'evidence' that he agrees with her negative self-view
Physical symptoms	Increasing tiredness and lethargy Muscular fatigue and weakness

What approaches could Diane's GP use to help Diane to feel less depressed and low?

Remember to include a range of different strategies, including cognitive approaches and behavioural changes.

Reminders: Depression in patients with physical illness

- One of the key aims is to increase recognition of depression in patients with chronic physical disease as it is often missed and is consequently under-treated
- Biological features of depression such as fatigue and lethargy may be confused with physical symptoms associated with a patient's medical problems
- Some drug treatments also *cause* depression as a side effect
- Depression is treatable in patients with chronic medical conditions and may include the use of antidepressant medication and psychological approaches

Anxiety in chronic illness

Anxiety is common amongst patients with physical disease. It is sometimes viewed as a normal response to physical illness, but prolonged or severe anxiety may indicate the presence of a co-existing anxiety disorder.

The diagnosis of anxiety in patients with medical conditions is complicated by the fact that a variety of medical conditions can mimic or directly cause anxiety. Many common medications may also cause anxiety symptoms.

Box 15.1:
Medical conditions mimicking or causing anxiety

- Thyrotoxicosis
- Hypoglycaemia
- Vertigo
- Anaemia
- Heart disease (may cause feelings of apprehension or dread)
- Poor pain control (e.g. in cancer)
- Alcohol or drug withdrawal
- Respiratory disease (e.g. asthma, COPD)
- Disorders of the central nervous system (including epilepsy and structural disorders)

Box 15.2:
Common drugs causing anxiety symptoms

- Bronchodilators – β_2 agonists, theophyllines
- Thyroxine
- Antidepressants (particularly SSRIs)
- Antihistamines
- Calcium-channel blockers (felodipine)
- Digoxin (at toxic levels)
- Anticonvulsants (e.g. carbamazepine)
- Antimicrobials (cephalosporins, ofloxacin, aciclovir)
- Non-steroidal anti-inflammatory drugs (indomethacin)
- Insulin (when hypoglycaemic)

Box 15.3:
Assessing anxiety levels in chronic illness

- Is the patient's medical condition associated with physical symptoms which they are interpreting *catastrophically*?
- Is the patient particularly aware of information about possible catastrophic or tragic outcomes of their condition?
- Is the patient using *safety behaviours* (aimed to prevent physical catastrophe) that are actually unhelpful?
- Is the patient experiencing physical symptoms related to anxiety? Is the patient misinterpreting the meaning of these symptoms, which might be making their anxiety worse?

Effective treatment can lead to direct improvement in anxiety symptoms and may also improve compliance with medical treatments. Failing to address anxiety symptoms can be associated with increased disability, increased use of health service resources and impaired quality of life (House & Stark, 2002).

The first stage is to make a full assessment of patients with a possible anxiety disorder associated with chronic ill-health (*Box 15.3*).

Approaches to managing anxiety in patients with medical conditions

- *Give adequate information*: giving patients detailed information about their condition may help to reduce anxiety. This includes information about the disease itself as well as about investigations, treatments and the hospitals or clinics where they will be cared for. Written information is often useful as anxious people may find it difficult to recall verbal discussions.

- *Preparation for unpleasant procedures*: giving detailed information about future procedures can reduce anxiety and fear of the unknown

- *Communicate effectively*: includes asking open questions to elicit and specifically address the patient's underlying health beliefs and fears and asking for feedback to prevent misunderstandings.

- *Give positive explanations for symptoms*: patients may find it easier to cope with symptoms if they understand why they arise

- *Give reassurance appropriately*: reassurance should be based on a discussion of the patient's underlying fears. Avoid giving excessive, 'blanket' reassurance, which may actually increase anxiety about health in the long-term.

- *Cognitive techniques*: discuss catastrophic and unrealistic nature of patients' thoughts, for example by using pie-charts to identify likely future outcomes for particular disorders. Use distraction to manage recurrent negative thoughts.

- *Behavioural approaches*: reduce unhelpful behaviours such as avoidance or safety behaviours, which increase anxiety and restrict patients' lives in the long-term. Use graded exposure to gradually return to normal, daily activities.

- *Medication*: consider use of medication where appropriate (e.g. beta-blockers, antidepressants)

Reminders: Anxiety in patients with physical illness

- Several medical conditions can mimic or cause anxiety and many common medications may also cause anxiety symptoms
- Failing to address anxiety symptoms can be associated with increased disability, increased use of health service resources and impaired quality of life
- Approaches to managing anxiety include clear communication, giving adequate information, using reassurance appropriately, challenging catastrophic thinking and reducing unhelpful behaviour such as avoidance

Introducing a psychological approach

Some patients with chronic physical disorders may not see the benefit or relevance in using a psychological approach to their problems. It can be helpful to reassure the patient that considering psychological or emotional aspects of problems does not involve *ignoring* physical symptoms or standard medical treatment for problems (e.g. continuing to seek adequate pain control using analgesia).

> "*Would it be useful to look at how to help you feel less anxious or low, as well as continuing to deal with the physical aspects of your problem?*"

It may also be helpful to discuss the benefits of improving mood:

> "*Some people find that physical symptoms become even worse if they feel anxious or low. It can be helpful to reduce these negative feelings, as well as treating your physical problems.*"

Box 15.4:
Strategies to increase acceptance of a psychological approach

- Engage the patient by beginning with questions about physical symptoms
- Acknowledge and summarize the patient's viewpoint
- Try to find some common ground
- Identify some genuine links between the patient's physical symptoms, thoughts, feelings and behaviour
- Ask to the patient to consider the benefits of including new perspectives for problems
- Emphasize that including psychological perspectives can be combined with standard medical approaches and treatment of their condition

Case example 15.4: Encouraging patients to accept a psychological approach

Michael is a 57-year old man with longstanding back and shoulder pain. He has tried a variety of different analgesic medications with little success. He has always been resistant to considering psychological or emotional aspects of his problems. In the following dialogue, Michael's GP begins the process of encouraging Michael to broaden his perspective of his problems.

Michael I'm so fed up with this pain. I've had it for so long and no-one has been able to help me with it.

GP How do you feel emotionally when you get the pain?

Michael [*Sounds annoyed*] I don't know what you mean. What I feel is really agonizing pain.

GP Did something about that question upset you?

continued

Michael I'm in terrible pain all the time and that's what I need to fix.
What's the point in going on about my emotions?

GP Some people find that being in constant pain makes them feel fed
up or angry. Sometimes, feeling strong emotions can actually make
pain even worse. It can sometimes be helpful to look at that side of
things as well as continuing to focus on your medical problems and
trying to improve your pain.

Michael Well I do feel extremely fed up and frustrated.

GP It sounds like you are quite angry that no-one has been able to help
you.

Michael Well, I keep going to different clinics and nothing makes any
difference. Half the doctors don't even listen to what I have to say.

GP Would it help if we spent some time today talking about how the
pain is affecting your life? That might help us find some new ways to
help.

Michael It probably won't help, but I'm prepared to give it a go.

GP I would like to talk about all the different aspects of your pain.
Could you begin by giving me an example of a time that the pain
was really severe and bothered you...?

**How could the consultation continue? What strategies could the GP
use to continue to encourage Michael to consider psychological,
behavioural and emotional aspects of his problems?**

Managing complex physical and emotional problems

Write a problem list

Patients with chronic disease often have a complex mix of physical and
emotional problems, which can be confusing and overwhelming for both
GP and patient. A useful way to make sense of this range of difficulties is to
write a *problem list*.

The first step is to write a list of all the patient's problems. This alone is
often a very useful exercise, which helps to direct the GP's attention to the
most important problems. The patient can be asked to prioritize these
problems and decide which ones to address first.

The next step is to explore the key problems in greater depth. This should
include an assessment of practical, physical, psychological and emotional
aspects of problems.

Making a list helps to make sense of a patient's problems and can make
difficulties seem more manageable. Sometimes patients will realize that
several problems on the list are related and that their list of difficulties is
not as long as they feared. By knowing what the exact problems are, it
becomes easier to identify which areas are most important, in order to
target the most helpful future interventions.

It is often helpful to spend time discovering exactly how specific difficulties or physical symptoms create problems for individual patients. Useful questions include:

"*What makes this a problem for you?*"

"*What is it about this that is troubling you the most?*"

It is sometimes useful to take a 'solution-focused' approach, by discussing what the patient would most like to achieve or change:

"*What would you most like to change?*"

"*If we could work together to improve something, what would this be?*"

Box 15.5:
Exploring
problem areas
in more depth

- What makes this a problem for this particular patient?
- Can you give me a recent example? What happened...?
- How do you think/feel/react? How do others react?
- What makes it better/worse (include cognitive/behavioural/situational factors)?
- Does it occur at particular times or in specific situations?
- Are there times that this is less of a problem for you? What are these?
- What particular beliefs does the patient hold about themselves, their illness, medical staff etc., which might be associated with this problem?

Case example 15.5: Using a problem list for patients with chronic disease

Jean is a 58-year old accounts clerk. She is overweight and has moderate hypertension. She has arthritis of both knees and is awaiting a left knee replacement. Her knees are very painful and she sometimes takes non-steroidal, anti-inflammatory medication, but has gastro-intestinal side effects. This limits how often she can take them.

Jean's problem list:
1. Arthritis in knees
2. Needs to lose weight
3. Husband had a heart attack last year
4. Problems at work
5. Feeling increasingly fed up and depressed

In the following dialogue, Jean and her GP discuss the impact of her worsening arthritis on her life.

GP   Which of these problems do you see as the most important to
      discuss first?

continued

Jean Well, life has become very difficult now that the arthritis in my knees has got so bad.

GP In what ways has this become a problem for you?

Jean I just can't do as much as I used to.

GP And what kinds of physical symptoms stop you...?

Jean I'm in a lot of pain. I also feel so tired nowadays.

GP Can you tell me what kinds of things that you are no longer doing, since you developed the arthritis? What did you used to do differently?

Jean I used to be very active. I was always out and about seeing friends. Now I hardly get out at all and I don't see my friends very often.

GP How does that make you feel?

Jean It makes me feel really fed up and down. Sometimes I get very angry about it.

GP I see. Can you tell me what makes you feel fed up? What goes through your mind when you feel that way?

Jean I think that my life is over. I'm only 58 but my life is so empty and meaningless now.

GP I understand. It must be very difficult to cope with the pain. I'd like to briefly summarize what you told me about your problems so far:

   You said that your arthritis is causing you a lot of pain and that you also feel very tired. Because of this, you are hardly able to get out and see your friends, which makes you feel very fed up and low, because you are thinking that "*My life is over. I'm only 58 but my life is empty and meaningless*". What do you make of all this? Is there anything you might be able to do to make any changes in this...?

Jean I can see how I really miss getting out of the house and seeing my friends. But it's so difficult with my arthritis.

GP It seems like you have got rather stuck. I wonder if there is any way that you might be able to make your life seem more enjoyable and worthwhile, even if you still continue to have the arthritis and pain?

Jean I hadn't really thought about it like that before. But I can see that it would make me feel better if I had more enjoyable things in my life. I will have to think about what I could still do.

GP That sounds like a really good idea. Perhaps we could make a list of suggestions...

continued

Jean and her GP repeated this discussion on several occasions, to construct the following table showing her most important problems:

Problem	Arthritis in knees	Need to lose weight	Husband had a heart attack last year
Physical symptoms associated	Pain, especially after walking Stiffness Tired and lethargic Poor sleep, tense	Makes arthritis worse Easily tired	Tense Poor sleep
Thoughts about problem	*"I'm in too much pain to enjoy life."* *"I can't do anything that I used to."* *"My life has really changed."*	*"Eating is my only pleasure in life"* *"I can't do any activity because of pain in my knees."* *"There's no point in trying – I will never manage to change"*	*"What if he has another one?"* *"I couldn't cope alone."* *"I am responsible for keeping him well."* *"He needs to constantly rest in order to protect his heart."*
Feelings	Frustrated Fed up/low	Guilty Low	Anxious Worried
Ways of behaving	Stopped walking to work Gradually cut down leisure activities Less social life	Try to 'be good' but frequent snacks Minimal activity/exercise	Frightened to leave him alone: *"What if he has another heart attack while I am out?"* Jean carries out most housework

By gradually building up an understanding of her problems, Jean is able to identify some simple ways to try to overcome some of these difficulties, including:

- Increasing time spent undertaking enjoyable activities or hobbies, despite the pain
- Gradually increasing gentle exercise such as swimming, which does not worsen knee pain
- Focus on a healthy eating plan, rather than extreme 'yo-yo' dieting regimes
- Encourage husband to take on more responsibility for jobs around the home (*"It is important to build up strength after a heart attack, rather than constantly resting"*). This may boost his self-esteem and gives Jean more time to focus on herself

Using a 'timeline' to understand the history of problems

For patients with complex, long-standing problems, it is often helpful to invest some time in going through their notes in detail and writing a summary of their key problems. This can save a great deal of time and effort in the long term. Gaining a better understanding of the patient and their history enables health professionals to make more informed decisions about medical care. The process may also reveal repetitive, unhelpful patterns of illness behaviour.

The summary should include:

- Key diagnoses
- Physical symptoms (acute exacerbations of the problem and deteriorations in physical health status)
- Hospital admissions
- Psychological and emotional difficulties
- Social and environmental factors (e.g. stopping work, illness in relatives)
- Referrals to secondary care (including outcome of referral)

The summary should also include information about any 'critical incidents', which may have triggered specific elements of emotional distress, such as:

- Reactions of other people to the problem
- Specific actions or statements by medical/nursing staff
- Media cover relating to own or similar medical problems
- Changes in medical/nursing care (e.g. change of medical practitioner)

Case example 15.6: Using a timeline

Summary of the medical history of a patient with chronic pelvic and abdominal pain:

Year	Age	Symptoms/life events	Referrals made	Investigations/ treatment	Diagnosis/ Outcome
1971	17	Lower abdominal pain (unhappy at school)	Surgical outpatients	Appendectomy	Normal
1975	21	Pregnant (boyfriend not supportive)	Gynaecology	Termination of pregancy	Nil
1980	26	Pelvic discomfort and heavy periods	Gynaecology	Dilatation and curettage	Possible endometriosis
1983	29	Pregnant	Obstetrics	High blood pressure during	Emergency caesarean delivery

continued

Year	Age	Symptoms/life events	Referrals made	Investigations/ treatment	Diagnosis/ Outcome
				pregnancy	
1986	32	Bereavement: death of mother and uncle in same year	Nil	None	Prolonged grief reaction – ?mild depression
1989	36	Recurrent pelvic pain and heavy periods Requests sterilization	Gynaecology	Sterilization	Pain worsens after surgery
1993	40	Divorce; daughter having difficulties at school	Nil	None	Anxious and stressed
1994	41	Heavy periods	Gynaecology	Hysterectomy	Develops urinary symptoms after surgery; pain persists
1999	45	Problems at work – (poor attendance due to ill-health); tribunal for unfair dismissal	Nil	None	Angry and low
1999	45	Abdominal pain worse	Gynaecology	Possible adhesions	Strong analgesic medication
2003	47	Poor housing conditions – social services involved Requests medical retirement from work	Social services	Nil	Moved to new flat after long delay
2004	48	Generalized muscle pains and tingling Fainted; complaining of memory loss	Neurology	Nil found; suggest rheumatology referral	Low dose amitriptyline
2004	48	Referred to rheumatology by neurologist	Rheumatology	Mild cervical spondylosis and arthritis	NSAIDs (cause heartburn)
2005	50	Chest pain and breathlessness	Cardiology	Nil found: ?anxiety-related	Beta-blockers

Reminders: Managing complex problems

- Writing a problem list is a useful way to make sense of complex physical and emotional problems and can be prioritized by patients into order of importance
- Exploration of specific problems identified by the list should involve assessing practical, physical, psychological and emotional aspects of problems.
- Writing a summary of complex, long-standing problems as a timeline may help GPs to make decisions about medical care and reveal repeated patterns of illness behaviour

Helping patients cope with uncertainty

Coping with uncertainty is an inevitable part of living with physical disorders. This is compounded by the medical system, which often involves long periods of waiting for information, test results and for hospital or other appointments. Some patients accept this uncertainty as inevitable. They are able to 'live for the moment' by focusing on what they *do* know rather than constantly worrying about what they do *not* know and are unable to control.

For other patients, uncertainty is associated with unbearable anxiety, hopelessness and fear. They may become preoccupied with negative, 'what if' thoughts about what might go wrong in the future. Some patients begin living their lives *'as if'* the worst has already happened.

For patients who are struggling to come to terms with uncertainty, it can be helpful to encourage them to face their fears, with a sensitive, open discussion about their underlying, anxiety-provoking thoughts.

> *"What is it about this that makes you feel so anxious? What thoughts are playing upon your mind?"*

This includes identifying an individual patient's specific fears. For example, a patient who fears dying may be afraid of future pain, or may be more concerned about the welfare of their loved ones after their death.

> *"If that did happen, what would be the worst part about it for you?"*
>
> *"What do you imagine happening that causes you so much distress?"*

Once the patient's specific, anxiety-provoking thoughts have been identified, the next stage may be to evaluate how realistic and helpful they are and to consider alternative possibilities, which provide a more balanced view of the future:

> *"Is this the most likely or realistic possibility? Is there any other way to view the situation?"*

Coping strategies for managing uncertainty

Identify coping strategies for dealing with potential problems

Spend time with patients discussing and planning how they could cope if the worst really did happen. Rather than simply focusing on the worst possible outcomes (*'What if...?'*), the patient can plan strategies for coping with each possibility (*'Then what...?'*).

Increase the patient's sense of control over life

Encourage patients to focus on aspects of their life that they genuinely have the power to change (e.g. how they spend their time each day), rather than continually focusing on areas they are powerless to control (e.g. what might happen in the future). This may include making helpful behavioural changes, such as increasing time spent with family and close friends, and other enjoyable or meaningful activities.

Acceptance of uncertainty as a normal part of life

Life is *always* filled with uncertainty. By focusing on the worst possible outcome and behaving *'as if'* this is the most likely outcome, or *'as if'* the worst has already happened, the patient's life becomes filled with negative thoughts, feelings and unhelpful behaviours, which simply compound their problems.

Case example 15.6: Managing uncertainty

Vanessa is a 45-year old woman who developed a malignant breast lump. The lump was successfully excised and subsequent scans revealed there was no evidence of spread of the disease. One year later, Vanessa is well, with no signs of a recurrence. However, she remains preoccupied and anxious that the cancer could return.

Vanessa I can't stop worrying about the future. I keep thinking, *"What if it comes back?"* or *"What if they can't treat it next time?"* I know I am well now and I am so grateful, but I just wish I could feel more relaxed about the future.

GP What would you need to feel more relaxed about the future?

Vanessa I just need to be sure that the cancer won't come back.

GP You would like to feel certain that the cancer will never come back?

Vanessa Yes, though I realize that is impossible. No-one can ever say that for sure.

GP I think you are probably right. No-one can ever be 100% sure about *anything* in the future. What is it about knowing for certain that would help you feel better?

Vanessa I would know that I could control things again.

GP What kinds of things would you like to have more control over?

Vanessa I could put my effort into continuing my life, by carrying on working, spending time with my children.

GP Are you concerned about losing control over these areas of your life?

Vanessa When I'm really anxious, I just think, *"I know it's all going to come back"* and I keep thinking about all these things that I will miss out on.

GP Are you doing these things less often than you used to?

continued

Vanessa I suppose I am. What's the point of putting effort into working or building up my life, if it will all be taken away by the cancer?

GP It sounds like you are saying that you sometimes worry about your future health and think, "*I know the cancer is going to come back,*" which makes you feel very anxious. And you react by reducing some activities, because it seems pointless to do them if you will develop cancer in the future. Is that right, do you think?

Vanessa Yes it is. I hadn't really thought of it like that before.

GP What do you make of it now? Are there any ways that this pattern is unhelpful to you?

Vanessa Well yes, because it means that I am cutting down the things that are actually really important to me.

GP All this worrying might actually be getting in the way of you doing the things that are important to you. Supposing the cancer did come back eventually. How would you want to look back at your life between now and then? Do you think you would want to have spent most of that time worrying about the future?

Vanessa No, not at all. I would probably want to think that I had enjoyed my life. I would want to have spent as much quality time as possible with my family. I wouldn't want to have spent all my time worrying about the future.

GP What could you do differently, that might help you more?

Vanessa I could try to focus on doing the things that really matter. Like spending time playing with my children and talking to my husband.

Reminders: Strategies for managing uncertainty

■ Remember that nothing in life can ever be certain
■ Identify the patient's specific anxiety-provoking thoughts and fears about the future. Evaluate whether these are a balanced or realistic way to view the situation.
■ Devise a 'Then what...?' plan, for coping with possible future problems
■ Increase the patient's sense of control by encouraging them to make changes in areas of their lives that they genuinely have the power to influence

Coping with changes in physical appearance

Many physical illnesses involve changes in appearance, which may cause a great deal of distress for some patients. In helping patients to come to terms with such changes, it is important to identify the *meaning* that the patient attributes to these changes. If patients associate their changes in appearance with a loss of their personal worth or value, they are likely to experience a loss of self-esteem and a lowering of mood. The negative perception may result from patients' beliefs about changes in the opinion of others or it may result from their view of themselves.

These negative self-views can be directly using cognitive restructuring techniques. Behavioural experiments are also an effective means of reinforcing new, more helpful beliefs.

Case example 15.7: Coping with changes in physical appearance

Reginald is a 76-year old widower who lives in a residential home. He has been diabetic for many years and suffers from vascular disease. He recently underwent a below-knee amputation. Reginald is well known for being a jovial man, who is well liked and sociable in the residential home. However, since his operation, he has become increasingly morose and withdrawn.

During a visit, Reginald's GP spends a few minutes discussing his change in mood since the amputation:

Thoughts	*"I look awful and others will not want to spend time with me."*
	"They will think I am not the same person anymore – not 'whole'."
Feelings	Sad
Behaviour	Avoids social situation
	Spends long hours alone in his room

Reginald's behavioural experiment planning chart:

What am I going to do? (What, where, when…?)	Attend the weekly in-house bingo evening. Invite a few old friends to join me.
What do I predict will happen?	My friends will react differently to me. They will seem uncomfortable and avoid looking at me. Some might make an excuse not to come or may sit elsewhere.
What problems might arise with this plan?	I might feel too tired or in pain to go.
How could these problems be overcome?	I will take my pain medication and have a brief nap during the afternoon beforehand.
What happened when I tried the experiment?	"Everyone seemed very pleased to see me. A couple of people said that I looked very 'well.' No one tried to avoid me. Several people made a point of coming over and saying they were pleased to see me."

What have I learned from this experiment?
"People don't necessarily think less of me for physical changes. Everyone changes in appearance with time for many reasons. This doesn't change me as a 'person'."

Reminders: Coping with changes in physical appearance

- Changes in appearance associated with some physical illnesses can cause a great deal of distress for patients
- If patients associate these changes with a loss of their personal worth or value, they are likely to experience a loss of self-esteem and a lowering of mood
- These negative self-views can be challenged cognitively or by using behavioural experiments to reinforce more helpful beliefs

Coping with unpleasant physical symptoms

People with chronic disease may experience a wide variety of physical symptoms, including pain, dizziness, tinnitus, gastro-intestinal symptoms, chronic cough or breathlessness. Some symptoms can be alleviated through the use of appropriate medication. However, many symptoms are difficult to eliminate entirely, and other symptoms may even be *caused* by the side effects of drug therapy.

It is often helpful for patients to develop effective strategies for coping with these unpleasant physical sensations. These may include:

- *Reduce self-focus:* reduce the amount of attention directed towards internal bodily processes. This can make physical sensations and symptoms seem less intrusive and unpleasant.
- *Distraction:* this can take the mind away from powerful unpleasant physical or emotional experiences
- *Activity scheduling:* increase activities which are enjoyable or which give life a sense of meaning
- *Exercise:* gradually build up exercise levels to increase fitness, improve mood and overcome fatigue and tiredness
- *Relaxation methods:* decrease background levels of anxiety and tension
- *Mindfulness* (see Chapter 7): may reduce the impact of unpleasant physical symptoms by encouraging patients to view them as simply one part of their experience
- *Identify and treat underlying emotional disorders:* e.g. depression or anxiety

Reminders: Coping with unpleasant physical symptoms

- People with chronic disease may experience a wide variety of physical symptoms, which cannot always be alleviated with medication
- Effective strategies for coping with unpleasant physical sensations include using distraction, activity scheduling, relaxation and exercise

Understanding chronic pain

Chronic pain is a syndrome of severe pain that persists in spite of medical treatment. Patients usually obtain only limited pain relief from medication and the presence of the pain often begins to dominate their lives. Patients with chronic pain frequently feel depressed, anxious about the future, experience a loss of enjoyment in their daily activities and may feel hopeless or helpless in the face of unremitting, intolerable pain.

The development of chronic pain is more strongly associated with *psychosocial variables,* such as emotional distress and social stressors, than with the degree of physical abnormality.

Box 15.6
Factors associated with the development of chronic pain

- Lack of care during childhood
- Family history of illness
- Dissatisfaction with work or unemployment
- High levels of psychological distress (e.g. presence of depression)
- Precipitating factors: injuries at work, other injuries (e.g. involvement in road traffic accident), other traumatic events

Typical thoughts in chronic pain

Patients with chronic pain typically hold a wide range of negative, unhelpful health beliefs, which are likely to result in unhelpful behavioural reactions. These may include:

"I must be completely free of pain to feel better"

"It is better to rest when I feel the pain"

"If my pain increases I must be doing permanent damage to myself"

"There is nothing I can do to control my pain"

Patients may also develop negative beliefs which lower their self-esteem:

"Having this pain means I am weak, incompetent or unlovable"

"Being unable to work means I am a failure"

They may also develop negative beliefs about the reactions of others:

"Others don't care about the agony I am experiencing"

"The doctor thinks I am making it up"

Patients with chronic pain may also hold highly negative views of the future, associated with feelings of hopelessness and depression:

"If I am feeling this much pain now, in the future it will be completely unbearable"

"I can hardly walk now so in a few years I will be in a wheelchair"

Feelings in chronic pain

Patients with chronic pain frequently experience severe emotional distress, including feelings of:

- Depression and hopelessness – likely to result in an increased perception of the severity of pain
- Anger
- Anxiety

Physical symptoms

Chronic pain is associated with many types of physical discomfort including headaches, back pain, muscular pain, arthritis, and abdominal or pelvic pain.

Other physical symptoms may also be associated with chronic pain syndrome, such as:

- Weakness and stiffness (often due to lack of activity)
- Anxiety-related symptoms, poor sleep
- Lethargy and fatigue
- Side effects of medication
- Weight gain – due to inactivity and over-eating

Behavioural changes

- Reduced activity – associated with beliefs that activity will exacerbate pain/underlying physical disorders
- Excessive resting
- Social isolation and withdrawal
- 'Pain behaviours', e.g. sighing, groaning, grimacing, using walking sticks, wheel chairs or other physical aids, such as cervical collars, complaining to others, limping and over-reliance on pain medications. These behaviours are often reinforced by the reactions of others (e.g. if a patient groans when moving, relatives may begin to take their arm or treat the individual in other ways that reinforce the 'sick role').

Environmental factors

It is important to spend time discussing relevant psychosocial factors that may influence the development and maintenance of chronic pain syndrome. This may include:

- Negative social impact of chronic pain (e.g. loss of job/social status, financial difficulties)
- Inter-personal factors (e.g. increased stress and pressure on families, altered relationships with others – 'invalid status')

- Concurrent environmental/social difficulties (e.g. dissatisfaction with work, relationship problems)
- Relevant past experiences of illness (in self and others)
- Attitudes and relationships with health professionals

Treatment aims in chronic pain

The aim of treatment in chronic pain is to shift the patient's focus from curing or eliminating pain to coping with the pain and improving their life, *despite the continued presence of pain*. It should involve a combined approach to treatment, which includes medical and psychological approaches. Any co-existing mood disorders, such as depression, should also be treated.

An appropriate initial goal for managing chronic pain within the primary care setting may simply be to improve the relationship between GP and patient. This may sometimes require the health professional to alter any of their own unhelpful thoughts or behaviour relating to the patient.

Using a pain diary

A pain diary can be used to record a patient's pain levels during a typical week. This can also be used to link pain to specific emotional or behavioural factors.

Box 15.7
Example of a pain diary

Date/time	What were you doing?	How severe was the pain? (0–100)	How did you feel at this time? (e.g. angry, sad, anxious)	What did you do to cope with the pain? How severe was it after this?
Tuesday 10 a.m.	Watching TV	70	Fed up	Took pain killers Went to sleep (50)
Wednesday 1 p.m.	Making lunch	80	Anxious	Took pain killers Phoned a friend (40)

Useful strategies for managing chronic pain include:

1. Cognitive strategies

- Identify, evaluate and 're-frame' negative thoughts about pain, 'dangers' of activity or negative views of the future
- Develop *acceptance*: learning to view pain as an unpleasant but potentially inevitable part of life, accepting that complete cure of pain is unlikely.

- Reduce catastrophic thinking about the impact of the pain ("*My life is completely ruined because of the pain*") or about future changes ("*Things will become unbearable in the future*")
- Distraction techniques: focus mind away from negative thoughts or pain

2. *Behavioural strategies*

Encourage patients to increase positive activity, by behaving 'as if' life was fulfilling and worthwhile, despite the pain. Exercise is particularly helpful, but must be built up gradually (pacing), in order to avoid the 'over-activity – under-activity' cycle. Here, patients overdo activity on days that they feel well and consequently feel exhausted for several days afterwards, which reinforces beliefs about the dangers of activity and exercise.

3. *Physical/medical strategies*

Effective pain management may require a multi-disciplinary approach, involving pain teams, primary care services and psychological support services. Relaxation techniques, such as deep breathing, progressive muscular relaxation, mediation and yoga, can also be useful to improve pain and sleep.

Case example 15.8: Understanding chronic pain

John is a 42-year old mechanic, who has experienced longstanding back and shoulder pain following an accident at work. He has not worked for over two years.

Thoughts	"*When I get the pain, it is better to rest otherwise I might do even more damage.*" "*I must be completely free of the pain before I can get on with my life.*" "*Nothing will ever improve for me.*"
Feelings	Sad, low Angry
Behaviour	Spends long hours lying on the sofa watching daytime TV Off work Increasingly isolated from his friends
Environment	8-year old son suffers from attention-deficit hyperactivity disorder – John finds it increasingly difficult to cope with him and tends to get very angry Marital difficulties – arguments with his wife Financial strain due to long-term unemployment

---

John's behavioural experiment planning chart:

Thought to test: "*Unless I rest when I get the pain I will cause more damage and make things worse.*"
Alternative view: *Pain is not dangerous. It is better to remain active*

What am I going to do? (What, where, when...?)	Try continuing activity despite the pain and see what happens. I will try doing something I enjoy for 20 minutes, such as one or two DIY jobs around the house.
What do I predict will happen?	I will experience agonizing pain after 5 minutes of activity. This will continue for at least a day afterwards.
What problems might arise with this plan?	I might feel too tired to do it. I might not be in the right mood.
How could these problems be overcome?	I will plan to do this even if I am not in the right mood and see what happens.
What happened when I tried the experiment?	"The pain continued but did not get worse. I was able to get a few things done and felt pleased with myself. My mood seemed a bit better afterwards."

What have I learned from this experiment?
"It can be a good thing to keep active. The pain may not be as bad as I expect. I can still get things done, even if I have the pain."

Reminders: Understanding chronic pain

- Chronic pain is a syndrome of severe pain, which persists in spite of medical treatment and is only partially alleviated by medication
- Patients with chronic pain often feel depressed, angry and anxious
- Treatment aims to improve a patient's ability to manage and cope with pain rather than to eliminate pain
- Understanding a GP's *own* responses may help to improve relationships with patients experiencing chronic pain

Chapter 16

Further reading and other useful CBT resources

References

N.B. References preceded by asterisks are not cited in the text

Understanding and improving GP consultations

Armstrong D (1996) Construct validity and GPs' perceptions of psychological problems. *Primary Care Psychiatry* **2**: 119–122.

Balint M (1964) *The Doctor, His Patient and The Illness.* Churchill Livingstone, Edinburgh.

Berne E (1964) *Games People Play.* Grove Press, New York.

Helman CG (1990) *Culture, Health & Illness.* Butterworth-Heinemann, Oxford.

*****Kurtz S, Silverman J, Draper J** (1998) *Teaching and Learning Communication Skills in Medicine.* Radcliffe Medical Press, Oxford.

Launer J (2002) *Narrative-based Primary Care: a Practical Guide.* Radcliffe Medical Press, Oxford.

Moral RR, Alamo MM, Jurado AM, Perula de Torres L (2001) Effectiveness of a learner-centred training programme for primary care physicians in using a patient-centred consultation style. *Family Practice* **18**(1): 60–63.

Neighbour R (1987) *The Inner Consultation.* Churchill Livingstone, Edinburgh.

Neighbour R (1992) *The Inner Apprentice.* Petroc Press, Newbury.

Pendleton D, Schofield T, Tate P, Havelock P (1984) *The Consultation: An Approach to Learning and Teaching.* Oxford University Press, Oxford.

Silverman J, Kurtz S, Draper J (1998) *Skills for Communicating with Patients.* Radcliffe Medical Press, Oxford.

Doctor–patient relationships/partnership/shared decision-making

Barry CA, Bradley C, Britten N, Stevenson F, Barber N (2000) Patients' unvoiced agendas in general practice consultations: qualitative study. *British Medical Journal* **320**: 1246–1250.

Becker MH, Maiman LA (1975) Sociobehavioural determinants of compliance with medical care recommendations. *Medical Care* **13**: 10–24.

*Britten N, Stevenson FA, Barry CA, Barber N, Bradley CP (2000) Misunderstandings in prescribing decisions in general practice: qualitative study. *British Medical Journal* **320**: *484–488.*

*Butler C, Pill R, Stott N (1998) Qualitative study of patients' perceptions of doctors' advice to quit smoking: implications for opportunistic health promotion. *British Medical Journal* **316**: 1878–1881.

Heath I (1999) Commentary: There must be limits to the medicalization of human distress. *British Medical Journal* **318**: 440.

*Mercer SW, Reilly D, Watt GC (2002) The importance of empathy in the enablement of patients attending the Glasgow Homeopathic Hospital. *British Journal of General Practice* **52**: 901–905.

Say R, Thomson R (2003) The importance of patient preference in treatment decisions – challenges for doctors. *British Medical Journal* **327**: 542–545.

Mental health/Psychiatry

American Psychiatric Association (APA) (1994) *Diagnostic and Statistical Manual of Mental Disorders,* 4th edn. American Psychiatric Association, Washington, DC.

Bracken P, Thomas P (2001) Post psychiatry: a new direction for mental health. *British Medical Journal* **322**: 724–727.

Craig TK, Boardman AP (1997) ABC of mental health: common mental health problems in primary care. *British Medical Journal* **314**,1609–1613.

Department of Health (DOH) (2001) *Treatment Choice in Psychological Therapies and Counselling.* Department of Health, London.

*Double D (2002) The limits of psychiatry. *British Medical Journal* **324**: 900–904.

*Hale A (1998) *ABC of Mental Health.* BMJ Books, London.

Kessler RC, McGonagle KA, Zhao S *et al.* (1994) Lifetime and 12-month prevalence of DSM-IIIR psychiatric disorders in the United States: results of the national comorbidity survey. *Archives of General Psychiatry* **51**: 8–19.

*Murray CJ, Lopez AD (1997) Regional patterns of disability-free life expectancy and disability adjusted life expectancy: global burden of disease study. *Lancet* **349**:1347–1352.

*Murray CJ, Lopez AD (1997) Alternative projections of mortality and disability by cause 1990-2020: global burden of disease study. *Lancet* **349**: 1498–1504.

Mental health in primary care

Kadam U, Croft P, McLeod J, Hutchinson M (2001) A qualitative study of patients' views on anxiety and depression. *British Journal of General Practice* **466**: 375–380.

*Marks JN, Goldberg DP, Hillier VF (1979) Determinants of the ability of general practitioners to detect psychiatric illness. *Psychological Medicine* **9**: 337–354.

Middleton H, Shaw I (2000) Distinguishing mental illness in primary care (editorial). *British Medical Journal* **320**: 1420.

*Pollock K, Grime J (2002) Patients' perceptions of entitlement to time in general practice consultations for depression: a qualitative study. *British Medical Journal* **325**, 687–692.

Thompson C, Kinmonth AL, Stevens L *et al.* (2000) Effects of a clinical-practice guideline and practice-based education on detection and outcome of depression in primary care: Hampshire Depression Project randomised controlled trial. *Lancet* **355**: 185–191.

Teaching and learning CBT and other approaches to mental health

*Blackburn IM, James IA, Baker C *et al.* (2001) The revised cognitive therapy scale (CTS-R): psychometric properties. *Behavioural and Cognitive Psychotherapy* **29**: 431–446.

David LS, Freeman GK (2006) Improving consultation skills using cognitive behavioural therapy: A new model for general practice. *Education for Primary Care* **17**(5): in press.

*Davidson O, King M, Sharp D, Taylor F (1999) A pilot randomised trial evaluating GP registrar management of major depression following brief training in cognitive-behaviour therapy. *Education in General Practice* **10**: 485–488.

*Friedberg R, Fideleo R (1992) Training in-patient staff in cognitive therapy. *Journal of Cognitive Psychotherapy* **6**: 105–112.

*Goldberg DP, Steele JJ, Smith C, Spivey L (1980) Training family doctors to recognize psychiatric illness with increased accuracy. *Lancet* **2**: 521–523.

*King M, Davidson O, Taylor F, Haines A, Sharp D, Turner R (2002). Effectiveness of teaching general practitioners skills in brief cognitive behaviour therapy to treat patients with depression: randomised controlled trial. *British Medical Journal* **324**, 927–986.

*Stopa L, Thorne P (1999) Cognitive-behavioural therapy training: Teach the formulation first. *Clinical Psychology Forum* **123**: 20–23.

General CBT theory and applications

*Beck AT (1976) *Cognitive Therapy and the Emotional Disorders*. International Universities Press, New York.

*Beck AT, Weishaar M (1986) Cognitive Therapy. In: *Cognitive Behavioural Approaches to Psychotherapy* (eds Dryden W, Golden W), pp. 61–92. Harper & Row, London.

*Beck J (1995) *Cognitive Therapy: Basics and Beyond*. Guildford Press, New York.

*Bennett-Levy J, Butler G, Fennell M, Hackmann A, Mueller M, Westbrook D (eds) (2004) *Oxford Guide to Behavioural Experiments in Cognitive Therapy*. Oxford University Press, Oxford.

Enright SJ (1997) Cognitive-behaviour therapy – clinical applications. *British Medical Journal* **314**: 1811–1816.

Greenberger D, Padesky CA (1995a) *Mind over Mood*. Guildford Press, New York.

Greenberger D, Padesky CA (1995b) *Clinician's Guide to Mind over Mood.* Guildford Press, New York.

*Hawton K, Salkovskis PM, Kirk J, Clark DM (eds) (1989) *Cognitive Behaviour Therapy for Psychiatric Problems. A Practical Guide.* Oxford University Press, Oxford.

*Neenan M, Dryden W (2002) *Cognitive Behaviour Therapy: An A-Z of Persuasive Arguments.* Whurr Publishers, London.

Padesky CA (1993) Schema as self-prejudice. *International Cognitive Therapy Newsletter* **5/6**: 16–17.

Padesky CA (2003) *Guided Discovery: Leading and Following (audiotape).* Centre for Cognitive Therapy, California.

Safran J, Segal Z (1990) *Interpersonal Processes in Cognitive Therapy.* Basic Books, New York.

Wills F, Sanders D (1997) *Cognitive Therapy. Transforming the Image.* Sage, London.

Case formulation in CBT

Padesky CA, Mooney KA (1990) Clinical Tip: Presenting the cognitive model to clients. *International Cognitive Therapy Newsletter* **6**: 13–14.

*Persons, J (1989) *Cognitive Therapy in Practice. A Case Formulation Approach.* W.W. Norton, New York.

Williams CJ, Garland A (2002) A cognitive-behavioural assessment model for use in everyday clinical practice. *Advances in Psychiatric Treatment* **8**(3): 172–179.

Heartsink

Butler CC, Evans M (1999) The heartsink patient revisited. *British Journal of General Practice* **49**(440): 230–233.

*Crutcher JE, Bass MJ (1980) The difficult patient and the troubled physician. *Journal of Family Practice* **11**: 933–938.

*Hodgson P, Smith P, Brown T, Dowrick C (2005) Stories from frequent attenders: a qualitative study in primary care. *Annals of Family Medicine* **3**: 318–323.

*Mathers N, Gask L (1995) Surviving the 'heartsink' experience. *Family Practise* **12**: 176–183.

Mathers N, Jones N, Hannay D (1995) Heartsink patients: a study of their general practitioners. *British Journal of General Practice* **45**: 293–296.

*O'Dowd TC (1988) Five years of heartsink patients in general practice. *British Medical Journal* **297**: 528–532.

Steinmetz D, Tabenkin H (2001) The 'difficult patient' as perceived by family physicians. *Family Practice* **18**(5): 495–500.

Mindfulness

Kabat-Zinn J (1990) *Full Catastrophe Living: Using the Wisdom of Your Mind and Body to Face Stress, Pain and Illness.* Delta, New York.

Kabat-Zinn J, Massio AO, Kristeller J *et al.* (1992) Effectiveness of a medita-tion-based stress reduction program in the treatment of anxiety disor-ders. *American Journal of Psychiatry* **149**: 936–943.

Kabat-Zinn J, Lipworth L, Burney R, Sellers W (1986) Four year follow-up of a meditation-based program for the self-regulation of chronic pain: treatment outcomes and compliance. *Clinical Journal of Pain* **2**: 159–173.

Kabat-Zinn J, Wheeler E, Light T *et al.* (1998) Influence of a mindfulness meditation-based stress reduction intervention on rates of skin clearing in patients with moderate to severe psoriasis undergoing phototherapy (UVB) and phytochemotherapy (PUVA). *Psychosomatic Medicine* **60**, 625–632.

Segal ZV, Williams JMG, Teasdale JD (2001) *Mindfulness-based Cognitive Therapy for Depression. A New Approach to Preventing Relapse.* Guildford Press, New York.

*****Teasale JD, Segal Z, Williams JMG, Ridgeway VA, Soulsby JM, Lau Ma** (2000) Prevention of relapse/recurrence in major depression by mindfulness-based cognitive therapy. *Journal of Consulting and Clinical Psychology* **68**: 615–623.

Problem-solving therapy

*****Mynors-Wallis L** (1996) Problem-solving treatment: evidence for effective-ness and feasibility in primary care. *International Journal of Psychiatry in Medicine* **26**(3): 249–262.

*****Mynors-Wallis L** (2005) *Problem Solving Treatment for Anxiety and Depression: A Practical Guide.* Oxford University Press, Oxford.

*****Mynors-Wallis LM, Gath DH, Day A, Baker F** (1995) RCT comparing problem solving treatment with amitriptyline and placebo for major depression in primary care. *British Medical Journal* **310**: 441–445.

Nezu AM, Nezu CM (1989) *Problem-solving Therapy for Depression: Theory, Research and Clinical Guidelines.* Wiley, New York.

Anxiety disorders

Beck AT, Emery G, Greenberg RL (1985) *Anxiety Disorders and Phobias: a Cognitive Perspective.* Basic Books, New York.

*****Butler G** (1999) *Overcoming Social Anxiety and Shyness.* Constable and Robinson, London.

Clark DM (1986) A cognitive model of panic. *Behaviour Research and Therapy* **24**: 461–470.

Kennerley H (1997) *Overcoming Anxiety.* Constable and Robinson, London.

National Institute for Clinical Excellence (NICE) (2004a) *Anxiety: Management of Anxiety in Primary, Secondary and Community Care.* Clinical guideline 23. NICE, London.

*****Salkovskis P, Clark D** (1993) Panic disorder and hypochondriasis. *Advances in Behaviour Research and Therapy* **15**: 23–48.

Wells A (1997) *Cognitive Therapy of Anxiety Disorders.* John Wiley and Sons, Chichester.

Depression/Low self-esteem

Beck AT, Rush AJ, Shaw BF, Emery G (1979) *Cognitive Therapy of Depression.* Guildford Press, New York.

Churchill R, Khaira M, Gretton V *et al.* (2000) Treating depression in general practice: factors affecting patients' treatment preferences. *British Journal of General Practice* **460**: 905–906.

*****Fennell M** (1999) *Overcoming Low Self-esteem.* Constable and Robinson, London.

*****Gilbert P** (2000) *Overcoming Depression.* Constable and Robinson, London.

*****Gill D, Hatcher S** (2000) Antidepressants for depression in medical illness. *Cochrane Database of Systematic Reviews* **4**: CD0001312.

Katon W, Schulberg H (1992) Epidemiology of depression in primary care. *General Hospital Psychiatry* **14**: 237–247.

National Institute for Clinical Excellence (NICE) (2004b) *Depression: Management of Depression in Primary and Secondary Care.* Clinical guideline 22. NICE, London.

Paykel ES, Scott J, Teasdale JD *et al.* (1999) Prevention of relapse in residual depression by cognitive therapy: a controlled trial. *Archives of General Psychiatry.* **56**: 829–835.

Scott C, Tacchi MJ, Jones R, Scott J (1997) Acute and one-year outcome of a RCT of brief cognitive therapy for major depressive disorder in primary care. *British Journal of Psychiatry* **171**: 131–134.

*****Ward E, King M, Lloyd M** *et al.* (2000) Randomised controlled trial of non-directive counselling, cognitive-behaviour therapy and usual general practitioner care for patients with depression I: Clinical effectiveness. *British Medical Journal* **321**: 1383–1388.

*****Wells KB, Stewart A, Hays RD** *et al.* (1989) The functioning and well-being of depressed patients. Results from the medical outcomes study. *Journal of the American Medical Association* **262**: 914–919.

*****Williams CJ** (2001) *Overcoming Depression: A Five Areas Approach.* Arnold, London.

Health anxiety and medically unexplained symptoms

Barsky AJ, Wyshak G, Klerman GL, Latham KS (1990) The prevalence of hypochondriasis in medical outpatients. *Social Psychiatry and Psychiatric Epidemiology* **25**: 89–90.

*****Bass C, May S** (2002) ABC of psychological medicine: Chronic multiple functional somatic symptoms. *British Medical Journal* **325**: 323–326/

*****Fitzpatrick R** (1996) Telling patients there is nothing wrong (editorial). *British Medical Journal* **313**: 311–312.

Kellner R (1985) Functional somatic symptoms and hypochondriasis. *Archives of General Psychiatry* **42**: 821–33.

*****Kuchemann C, Sanders D**. *Understanding Health Anxiety: A Self-Help Guide for Sufferers and Their Families.* Oxford University Press (Oxuniprint), Oxford.

*****McDonald IG, Daly J, Jelinek JM, Panetta F, Gutman JM** (1996) Opening Pandora's box: the unpredictability of reassurance by a normal test result. *British Medical Journal* **313**: 329–332.

Raine R, Haines A, Sensky T, Hutchings A, Larkin K, Black N (2002) Systematic review of mental health interventions for patients with common somatic symptoms: can research evidence from secondary care be extrapolated to primary care? *British Medical Journal* **325**:1082.

*Ring A, Dowrick C, Humphris G, Salmon P (2004) Do patients with unexplained physical symptoms pressurize general practitioners for somatic treatment? A qualitative study. *British Medical Journal* **328**: 1319–1320.

*Ring A, Dowrick CF, Humphris GM, Davies J, Salmon P (2005) The somatizing effect of clinical consultation: what patients and doctors say and do not say when patients present medically unexplained physical symptoms. *Social Science Medicine* **61**(7): 1505–1515.

*Salkovskis P, Bass C (1997) Hypochondriasis. In: *Science and Practice of Cognitive Behaviour Therapy* (eds Clark D, Fairburn C). Oxford University Press, Oxford, pp. 313–40.

*Sanders D (1996) *Counselling for Psychosomatic Problems*. Sage, London.

Speckens AE, Van Hemert AM, Spinhoven P, Hawton KE, Bolk JH, Rooijmans HG (1995) Cognitive behavioural therapy for medically unexplained physical symptoms: a randomised controlled trial. *British Medical Journal* **311**: 1328–1332.

Warwick H, Salkovskis P (1989) Hypochondriasis. In: *Cognitive Therapy in Clinical Practice: an Illustrated Casebook* (eds Scott J, Mark J, Williams G, Beck AT). Routledge, London, pp. 78–102.

Warwick HM, Clark DM, Cobb AM, Salkovskis PM (1996) A controlled trial of cognitive-behavioural treatment of hypochondriasis. *British Journal of Psychiatry* **169**: 189–195.

Psychological aspects of physical disease

*Bass C, May S (2002) ABC of psychological medicine: Chronic multiple functional somatic symptoms. *British Medical Journal* **325**: 323–326.

House A, Stark D (2002) ABC of psychological medicine: Anxiety in medical patients. *British Medical Journal* **325**, 207–209.

*Kenardy J (2003) Review: cognitive behaviour therapy and behaviour therapy may be effective for back pain and chronic fatigue syndrome, and antidepressants may be effective for irritable bowel syndrome. *Evidence Based Medicine* **8**(3): 88.

*Mayou R, Farmer A (2002) Functional somatic symptoms and syndromes. *British Medical Journal* **325**: 265–268.

Peveler R, Carson A, Rodin G (2002) ABC of psychological medicine: Depression in medical patients. *British Medical Journal* **325**: 149–152.

*Thomas E, Silman AS, Croft PR, Papageorgiou AC, Jayson MIV, Macfarlane GJ (1999) Predicting who develops chronic low back pain: a prospective study. *British Medical Journal* **318**: 1662–1667.

*Van Tulder M, Ostelo R, Vlaeyen J, Linton S, Morley S, Assendelf W (2000) Behavioural treatment for chronic low back pain. *Cochrane Database of Systematic Reviews* **2**: CD002014.

*White C (2001) *Cognitive Behaviour Therapy for Chronic Medical Problems*. John Wiley and Sons, Chichester.

Further reading for health professionals

See also the references section above for further reading on specific topics.

Also remember that many self-help books/leaflets (see lists below) offer a highly useful, readable and practical introduction to CBT for health professionals, as well as patients.

Cognitive Therapy: Basics and Beyond by Judith Beck (published by Guildford Press)
   Good introduction to CBT.

Cognitive Therapy of Depression by Aaron T. Beck (published by Guildford Press)
   The original CBT text. Still highly useful and relevant.

Cognitive Therapy: an Introduction by Diana Sanders and Frank Wills (published by Sage Publications Ltd)
   Another useful introductory overview of CBT

Clinician's Guide to Mind Over Mood by D. Greenberger and C.A. Padesky (published by Guildford Press)
   Useful adjunct to the self-help book *Mind Over Mood* by the same authors. Sets out ways of incorporating self-help approaches for patients into a variety of clinical settings.

Cognitive Behaviour Therapy for Psychiatric Problems. A Practical Guide by K. Hawton, P.M. Salkovskis, J. Kirk and D.M. Clark (eds) (published by Oxford University Press)
   Useful overview of common psychiatric problems using CBT, if somewhat dry style of writing. May be a little dated.

Oxford Guide to Behavioural Experiments in Cognitive Therapy by J. Bennett-Levy, G. Butler, M. Fennell, A. Hackmann, M. Mueller and D. Westbrook (eds) (published by Oxford University Press)
   Useful and practical guide to understanding and implementing behavioural experiments in CBT

Training for health professionals

British Association of Behavioural and Cognitive Psychotherapies (BABCP)

BABCP (www.babcp.com; tel: 01254 875277) is a multi-disciplinary interest group for professionals involved in theory and practice of CBT. The website offers a very useful resource with information about:

* CBT training and events throughout the UK
* Contains printable brief patient leaflets
* Provides details of accredited CBT practitioners – searchable by area – patients can self-refer to private therapists

Other training events

Dr Lee David runs workshops for GPs and other primary care health professionals on using the '10-minute CBT' approach outlined in this book. For further details on upcoming events or to arrange a training event in your area, e-mail her on: cbm.training@gmail.com or look at www.10minuteCBT.co.uk. (The website also contains several useful printable CBT leaflets for patients.)

Self-help publications for patients

Books

Mind Over Mood by Dennis Greenberger and Christine Padesky (published by Guildford Press)
> Extremely useful CBT-based self-help book. Outlines CBT principles applicable to a wide variety of clinical problems. **Highly recommended**.

Overcoming Depression by Paul Gilbert; *Overcoming Low Self-esteem* by Melanie Fennell; *Overcoming Anxiety* by Helen Kennerley; *Overcoming Panic* by Derrick Silove; *Overcoming Social Anxiety* by Gillian Butler; *Overcoming Anger and Irritability* by William Davies ('Overcoming' series published by Constable & Robinson)
> Useful and reasonably priced series of short books written by UK cognitive therapists. Specific to different clinical problems. **Highly recommended**.

Overcoming Depression and *Overcoming Anxiety* by Christopher Williams (published by Hodder Arnold)
> Two self-help titles for patients taking a 'five-areas approach' to overcoming problems using CBT principles. Use jargon-free language. Each book is categorized into several workbooks, looking at specific aspects of problems.

The Feeling Good Handbook by David Burns (published by Penguin Books Ltd)
> Another good general CBT-based self-help book. Some may find the style of the book somewhat 'American'.

Feel the Fear and Do it Anyway by Susan Jeffers (published by Rider Publications)
> Great 'lay book' for coping with anxiety and fear in a variety of situations.

Manage Your Mind by Gillian Butler and Tony Hope (published by Oxford Paperbacks)
> This book takes a CBT approach to both personal and professional (work-related) problems.

Full Catastrophe Living: Using the Wisdom of Your Mind and Body to Face Stress, Pain and Illness by Jon Kabat-Zinn (published by Piatkus books)
> An interesting introduction to mindfulness-based stress reduction.

Leaflets

Oxford Cognitive Therapy Centre (www.octc.co.uk or 01865 223986) publish a variety of extremely useful and succinct CBT-based leaflets containing detailed explanations and advice on coping strategies for various disorders. These are highly recommended and can be purchased by practices or individual patients. Includes the following titles:

Building Self-esteem by Helen Jenkins and Melanie Fennell

Controlling Anxiety by Melanie Fennell and Gillian Butler

Managing Anxiety by Gillian Butler

Managing Depression by David Westbrook

Managing Obsessive-compulsive disorder by David Westbrook and Norma Morrison

Overcoming Social Anxiety by Gillian Butler

Understanding Health Anxiety by Christine Kuchemann and Diana Sanders

Understanding Panic by David Westbrook and Khadija Rouf

Understanding your Reactions to Trauma by Claudia Herbert

N.B. OCTC also host a variety of interesting CBT training events

Relaxation audiotape/CD

Simple relaxation tape which guides the listener through a series of relaxation exercises (progressive muscular relaxation) Available from OCTC (details above).

How to Relax by Helen Kennerley

Index